BABY BOOMERS' GUIDE
TO HEALTHY AGING

Baby Boomers' Guide To Healthy Aging

Bob Murphy

ROBERT D. REED PUBLISHERS • SAN FRANCISCO, CA

Robert D. Reed Publishers
750 La Playa Street, Suite 647
San Francisco, CA 94121
Phone: 650/994-6570 • Fax: -6579
E-mail: 4bobreed@msn.com
www.rdrpublishers.com

Book Design by Marilyn Yasmine Nadel

ISBN: 1931741166
Library of Congress Control Number: 2002102611

Produced and Printed in the United States of America

To my parents

CONTENTS

GLOSSARY OF TERMS .ix

Chapter 1   ALL OF US ALIENS 13

Chapter 2   THE BUILDING BLOCKS OF THE TEMPLE:
             THE MOLECULES OF LIFE 31

Chapter 3   CONSUMED BY A SLOW FIRE 50

Chapter 4   MATTERS OF THE HEART 83

Chapter 5   CONFRONTING THE CRAB 116

Chapter 6   THE TROUBLE WITH AGING BONES 150

Chapter 7   THE AGING BRAIN .181

Chapter 9   FINDING THE NOBILITY WITHIN 209

             INDEX 219

GLOSSARY OF ABBREVIATIONS

-OH(s)	hydroxyl group(s)
-SH(s)	sulfydryl group(s)
A	adenine or australopithecus
A.aferensis	Australopithecus Aferensis
AAP	amyloid precursor protein
ACTH	adrenocorticotrophic hormone
Ach	acetylcholine
AD	Alzheimer's disease
ADP	adenosine diphosphate
AGE(s)	advanced glycation end products
AIDS	acquired immune deficiency syndrome
ALS	amyotrophic lateral sclerosis
AMP	adenosine monophosphate
APC(s)	antigen presenting cell(s)
ATP	adenosine triphosphate
Ar. A	arachidonic acid
B-cell	B- lymphocyte
BMD	bone mineral density (a measurement of bone density)
BMI	body mass index
BP	blood pressure
C	cytosine
CAT	catalase
CH_4	methane
CHD	coronary heart disease
CHO(s)	carbohydrate(s)
CMV	cytomegalovirus
CNS	central nervous system
CO_2	carbon dioxide
CSF	cerebro-spinal fluid
CT	connective tissue
CoA	coenzyme A

DHA	docosahexenoic acid
DHEA(S)	dehydroepiandrosterone (sulfate)
DNA	deoxyribonucleuc acid
EBP	eosinophil basic protein
EDRF	endothelium-derived relaxation factor
EPA	eicosapentenoic acid
ETC	electron transport chain
FA(s)	fatty acid(s)
FAD	flavin adenine dinucleotide (oxidized) form
$FADH_2$	flavin adenine dinucleotide (reduced) form
FFM	fat free mass
Fe^{2+}	ferrous ion
Fe^{3+}	ferric ion
G	guanine
GLA	gamma linolenic acid
GPX	glutathione peroxidase
GP(s)	general practitioner(s)
GSH	reduced glutathione
GSSG	oxidized glutathione
H	homo or helicobacter
H. pylori	Helicobacter pylori
H_2O water	
H_2O_2	hydrogen peroxide
HCl	hydrochloric acid
HDL	high-density lipoprotein
HIV	human immuodeficiency virus
HLA	human leukocyte antigen
HRT	hormone replacement therapy
Hb	hemoglobin
Hg	mercury
IAAT	intra-abdominal adipose tissue
IDDM	insulin dependent diabetes mellitus
IL	interleukin

INF	interferon
Ig(E)	immunoglobulin (E)
LA	linoleic acid
LAB	lactic acid bacteria
LBM	lean body mass
LDL	low density lipoprotein
LNA	linolenic acid
MAS	milk-alkali syndrome
MT	melatonin
Mg	magnesium
N-3	omega-3 (fatty acid)
N-6	omega-6 (fatty acid)
NAD^+	nicotinamide adenine dinucleotide (oxidized)
NADH	nicotinamide adenine dinucleotide (reduced)
NFT	neurofibrillary tangles
NH_3	ammonia
NIDDM	non-insulin dependent diabetes mellitus
NK	cell natural killer lymphocyte
NP	neuritic plaques
NSAID(s)	non-steroidal anti-inflammatory drug(s)
O_2	oxygen
O_3	ozone
OA	osteoarthritis
OC	oral contraceptive (pill)
PD	Parkinson's disease
PGI_2	prostacyclin I2
PMS	premenstrual syndrome
PNI	psychoneuroimmunology
PUFA	polyunsaturated fatty acid
RNA	ribonucleic acid
ROS	radical oxygen species

SCFA	short chain fatty acids
SLE	systemic lupus erythematosus
SMC(s)	ooth muscle cell(s)
SO_2	sulfur dioxide
SOD	superoxide dismutase
SaFA(s)	saturated fatty acid(s)
Se	selenium
T	thymine
T-cell	T-lymphocyte
TABP	Type A Behavior Pattern
TH cells	T-helper cells
TNF	tumor necrosis factor
U	uracil
UFA	unsaturated fatty acid
UK	United Kingdom
USA	United States of America
UV	ultraviolet
WHR	waist to hip ratio
c-FA(s)	cis-fatty acid(s) or cis- isomer of
cm	centimeter
g	gram(s)
iu	international units
kJ	kilojoules
kcal	kilocalories
kg	kilograms
km	kilometer
mL	milliliter(s)
mm	millimeter(s)
mol	mole
mtDNA	mitochondrial DNA
mya	million years ago
o-LDL	oxidized-LDL
t-FA(s)	trans-fatty acid(s) or trans- isomer

CHAPTER 1

ALL OF US ALIENS

Life has its own hidden forces which you only discover by living
P. R. Regamey, *Poverty*

Now that we have reached, or are nearing, the big 50, it may be time for some reflection. We have each of us been on a journey. A journey of self-discovery, as much as anything else. That is what life is really about, self-discovery. Let us now permit ourselves, a little self-indulgence and reflect upon our achievements.

We have already achieved much! We survived our teenage and early twenties. Many of us had children, and survived them too, although there were times when we were sure that someone would not. A large number of us went to the Vietnam War. Sadly, many of our number did not return. Others survived the war, but came home with bits missing, physical, mental, spiritual, or all of the above. Still others, survived the war, but did not survive the homecoming.

We, each of us, in our own way, have had our challenges. Each of us has his or her own story. This generation has collectively faced almost all the challenges that the human experience can offer, and is now fifty-ish. But our story is far from over in that there are still many pages to be written. It can be a successful story with a happy ending.

Ahead of us, large and threatening, are two more challenges. The big ones: aging and dying. It is natural for us to worry about aging because throughout our lives we had thought it had no connection with us. Being old was something that others experienced. But now things are different for us. Sometimes now, when the wind and rain pounded at the windows, and we were feeling a bit low, we find ourselves wondering: "*Is it all going to be downhill from here? Are we now going to slip inevitably into the decay and degeneration, which we have seen in previous generations?*"

For most of our lives, we have been lucky, living our youth in the 50s, 60s and early 70s, when, for the most part, at least in Western countries, it was a time of affluence, and possibly the only time in history when capitalism really worked. Are the gods now demanding that dues to be paid, even by us, The Lucky Generation? Is this our penance for having been so fortunate in so many other respects?

Old age does not necessarily mean degeneration into illness and incapacity. We can be vital and active well into our old age, and mentally alert too. The degeneration that we have seen in previous generations is not inevitable. It was largely the result of poor maintenance. If you want your equipment to last, to look good, and to work well, you have to look after it. The reason for this book is so that we can all think about how to do that.

The fact that we do tend to degenerate during our aging is largely connected with our difficulty dealing with the highly reactive element oxygen. Oxygen is, to some degree at least, alien to our systems. This is because most of the cells of which our bodies are made, evolved before oxygen was common in the atmosphere. In order to tell this story, I must tell you the story of the beginning of life, because it was during this epoch that our ambivalent relationship with oxygen began.

The absolute beginning of you and me and everything, took place in another part of the universe, many millions, perhaps even billions of years ago, and trillions of kilometers from earth. That is where and when you began. You are already ancient! All the atoms of which you are made, except hydrogen, were founded and tempered inside a star, at a temperature of tens of millions of degrees Celsius, maybe millions of light years away, and perhaps billions of years ago. They were then cast into space, either as part of the outer shell of a decaying red, giant star, or possibly in a gigantic stellar explosion, called a supernova. All of the atoms in your body had this antique and dramatic birth.

We are the children of the universe. Our nursery was the stars. We are an aspect of the universe that has developed self-awareness.

We are part of the great parade of living things, the process by which the universe has developed consciousness. So, how did this happen? How did we happen? To answer this, we have to go far back in time.

It is thought that life on the earth began about 3.5 billion years ago, at a time when the young earth was a very hostile place. The earliest fossils found of life on earth date to this period. One called *The Archean Epoch.* Life may have existed a little before this period, but not much before, since then the earth would then have been too hostile too hostile to support life.

At this time, Earth was vastly different from what it is today. If we were to revisit it, we would need a highly protective and self-contained environment, like the ones astronauts use in space, because the surface would be unsuitable for advanced life, such as ourselves. The atmosphere that we would see would be a thick smog, like a yellow-brown blanket, filling the sky and blocking out the sun for most of the day, and composed of the poisonous gases, carbon dioxide (CO_2), sulfur compounds, and sulfur dioxide, as well as photochemical smog. Water vapor, dust and ash, from the many volcanic eruptions, would also fill the atmosphere, the dust and ash causing its opacity and color. The surface temperature would be just below 100 degrees Celsius. The seas then condensing from the atmosphere would be close to boiling point.

There are three reasons why Earth was so hot at this time. Firstly, Earth's hot interior, the magma, fueled by its radioactivity, had not cooled. Secondly, without a protective atmosphere of oxygen (O_2) to burn meteors upon entry, it was pounded relentlessly by large meteors and asteroids and the impact from these would itself heat the surface. Thirdly, the dense pall of CO_2 and water vapor created an insulating layer would trap heat in the lower atmosphere. This is of course, what today we call *the Greenhouse Effect.* This greenhouse effect however, was far more efficient than anything that humans are likely able to manufacture.

To make matters worse, Earth had not by then developed its protective shields of ozone, which today helps to filter out some of the sun's intensity, and ultraviolet (UV) radiation. In this inhospitable nursery of life, the sun, although hidden by the thick clouds for long periods, would still heat the atmosphere, and this heat would dissipate only slowly.

At this time, the Earth was of course, barren. Plants and animals had not yet evolved. Everywhere, our world was craggy, rocky, and hilly. Volcanoes pierced the cloudy atmosphere with their pyrotechnics, and spewed red-hot rivulets of larva down their slopes, and for long distances. Hot mud-pools bubbled and gurgled. It was a hot and humid, wet world. Daytime was a perpetual twilight. The intense heat produced turbulence in the atmosphere, and storms in these murky skies were frequent.

Barbed tongues of lightning arced and forked though the mustard-brown gestational sky, parting its turgid viscosity for a moment, but only a moment. The world was a hot dark place, as hot as an oven, an oven in which the stuff of life was being incubated. Somewhere in the shallows of the warm seas, or in some primordial mud-pools, under the brown and brooding sky, the elements of life, of you and me, were being assembled.

Of course, ovens are not much use without a recipe. Like any other recipe, the recipe of life needed certain ingredients. The recipe was in the mind of the Universe. The ingredients needed were: some energy, in the form of sunlight and lightning, and some catalysts.

Catalysts are naturally occurring substances that speed up chemical reactions. Both of these were already here, but, more than anything else, in order to evolve life on this planet, the Universe needed the ingredients of life simple organic molecules. Organic molecules are built from carbon, hydrogen, O_2 , nitrogen and phosphorous. It seems these molecules did not arise on the surface of Earth itself. They may have come from deep underground, but more than likely though, impacting asteroids, meteors and comets, from somewhere else in space, brought them.

Since these building blocks are our building blocks, you could say that each of us can trace his or her ancestry back to some other part of the solar system, perhaps some other part of the galaxy. We are all immigrants.

It was accepted for most of the 20th century that these primary organic molecules of life originated on the surface of the earth. This idea was first suggested by a Russian biochemist Alexksandr Oparin in the 1920s. He declared that the early atmosphere of Earth was mostly methane, ammonia, water and hydrogen.

In the 1950s, Stanley Miller, a graduate student at the University of Chicago, together with Nobel Prize laureate, Harold Urey, conducted a classic and elegant experiment designed to prove that amino acids could spontaneously self-assemble from the primordial atmosphere.

They took the gases methane, ammonia, hydrogen and steam, the ones Oparin had said composed the early atmosphere, and put them in a glass vessel. They then discharged an electric current into this mixture. This discharge represented some early energy input, perhaps like a lightning strike in the primordial atmosphere. What they then found, to their great excitement, was that the inside of this vessel had become thickly coated with amino acids. Since it is known that amino acids are fundamental building blocks of proteins, and that the formation of proteins is a necessary prerequisite for life, Miller and Urey believed they had discovered the mechanism by which life might have evolved on the young Earth.

What was wrong with this experiment was the assumption. Today, we know that the most abundant gas in the early atmosphere was CO_2. This gas is by far the most abundant gas on Mars and Venus, our two nearest neighbors, but today it represents a very small percentage of our atmosphere (although one that is rising as we burn fossil fuels). In the atmosphere of early Earth however, CO_2 was much more common. What has happened to it since is described by geologists as *The Carbon Cycle* whereby the CO_2 in the atmosphere became dissolved in seawater, combining with dissolved calcium, and precipitating out, as calcium carbonate, or limestone. Over the eons, much of the atmosphere's CO_2 was converted limestone. Today, there is 100,000 times more CO_2 in limestone than in the atmosphere.

Ancient CO_2 is today also locked up in fossil fuels, which we are now burning, and thereby reversing the process. In using fossil fuels, and returning CO_2 to the atmosphere, we are making today's atmosphere resemble the atmosphere of 3.5 billion years ago. This will not kill the planet. The planet has been through all this before and will take it in its stride. The same or similar mechanisms for fixing atmospheric carbon will begin again, but it may be too late for humans.

The Greenhouse Effect has always existed on this planet since the first volcanic explosions put CO_2 into the atmosphere. Indeed, without *The Greenhouse Effect* life would probably not exist on this planet, as the average surface temperature would be -18 degrees Celsius instead of the current balmy +15 degrees.

Back to Miller and Urey's experiment, if you repeat it, with CO_2 present in the proportion that is believed to have been present in the primordial atmosphere, it doesn't work! No amino acids, no building blocks of life are produced. So if the early organic molecules necessary for the evolution of life were like this, where did they come from? The answer is: from out there! Star Trek territory! They came from outer space, of course. Thus, in a very real sense, we are, all of us, aliens.

How can we be so sure that this was what happened, you might ask, since we rarely get an asteroid impact today? In terms of visiting asteroids and meteors, the young Earth was a much livelier place than it is now. Firstly, the inner solar system itself was far more active than today, when our planet is located in a quiet little cul-de-sac of the solar system. Three to four billion years ago it was in the path of a planetary six-lane highway. The inner planets, including Earth, had themselves just formed. One of the processes by which the planets form is by accretion of material within from within the solar system.

In this way, Earth and other planets were built, by condensation from interstellar gas, and by the gradual accumulation of stuff from the neighborhood.

We do know that amino acids, and other organic molecules, are in meteors. We also know that comets, such as Haley's, also contain organic molecules, and sometimes they, too, collide with Earth. Indeed it is likely, that it was a very large comet that hit Tunguska, in Siberia on June 30, 1908. So it seems likely indeed, that the early organic molecules needed for the beginnings of life were brought here by impaction from meteors, asteroids, and comets.

After a time, these early organic molecules would gradually build up, increasing with every impact event. At the same time, the radioactive material that had been fueling the heating of the magma began to decay. So, with time, two things important for life beginning occurred simultaneously the gradual cooling of the planet, and the enrichment of its surface with organic molecules.

We are the stuff of the stars; the very atoms of which we are made were manufactured in the centers of stars. The Universe, of which we are a part, needs creatures like us to evolve and flourish, because we provide a way by which she can develop self-awareness.

We are the Universe's way of contemplating itself. We are no more, and certainly no less, than a creative fragments of a Universe. Mother seeded this planet with what was needed to enable life to develop.

Once here, these simple organic molecules, under the influence of lightning and ultraviolet light, reacted to form other organic molecules, such as hydrogen cyanide and formaldehyde. These were later transmuted, through the alchemy of the laws of science, into amino acids, sugars, and the purine and pyrimidine bases required to make nucleotides.

To understand how life happened here, how Star Stuff, to use Carl Sagan's lovely expression, become the stuff of life, we first must understand a little about the chemistry of life, and the basic building blocks from which all life is made. That is, we need to learn a little biochemistry.

The most basic organic molecules, those that would be needed if life were to start, are amino acids, and these were probably the first biological chemicals created. They are molecules necessary for the construction of proteins. Proteins are very long strings of amino acids, all bound together through peptide bonds, and folded in a specific three-dimensional way. The individual strings, and a protein can contain several, are called polypeptides.

Proteins are vital for life. They are necessary as enzymes or biological catalysts. The chemical reactions needed for biology would not have occurred without enzymes, or would have happened too slowly to be useful. Enzymes increase the rate at which biological chemicals react with each other, by a million times. Advanced organisms also use proteins to transport necessary things around the body. Proteins enable the body to move, and to defend itself against infection.

Many of the body's messengers, hormones, are amino acid based, and are carried on circulating proteins. All the proteins in all living things from bacteria to humans are constructed from only 20 amino acids.

For life to develop, one other simple organic molecule was needed: the nucleotide. It has three components joined by the chemistry of life, a nitrogen-containing base, a sugar, and one or more phosphate groups.

Two polymers of nucleotides are vitally important for life. These are DNA (deoxyribonucleic acid) and RNA (ribonucleic acid). We call them polymers because they are composed of many nucleotide units joined together (poly a word derived from the Greek element polys means many). DNA is a polymer of deoxyribonuceotide units. The sugar in the deoxyribonucleotide is deoxyribose. The deoxy prefix indicates that this sugar lacks an oxygen atom normally present in ribose.

It is generally believed that RNA was the first of these two nucleic acids to be created by the Universe. DNA and RNA work together, building proteins, which form the structural elements of all life forms. DNA does not directly synthesize proteins, but acts like a manager, copying the genetic code, or pattern, of the required protein into RNA. It is these patterns that are used as templates for protein synthesis.

What makes nucleotides distinctive, however, is the base. As we saw, a nucleotide consists of a base, a sugar, and a phosphate. In DNA there are only four kinds of bases. These are adenine (A), guanine (G), thymine (T), and cytosine (C). RNA, like DNA, is composed of nucleotides, but it differs in two respects: the sugar in RNA is ribose, instead of deoxyribose, and the base thymine (T) is replaced with uracil (U). It was necessary for DNA to have a slightly different set of bases so that changes to the all-important genetic code which it carries, can't be altered by accident. This might have happened if DNA had identical bases to those in RNA.

As well as transmitting genetic code and organizing the synthesis of proteins, nucleotides can carry energy. Adenosine triphosphate (ATP) is a nucleotide that does this. We will discuss this high energy phosphate compound later. Its function is as a source of energy for cell chemistry.

Another clever trick of polynucleotides is to catalyze reactions. These can be reactions involving other polynucleotides. Catalysts make reactions occur faster. Enzymes, which are biological catalysts, lower the barriers that block chemical reactions, but, for simplicity, let's say that they speed them up.

Let's look at the RNA in the primordial mud-pool. There are many forms of RNA. Some can act as catalysts, 'speeding up' the joining together of bases to form new RNA molecules, while still others catalyze the breaking of these bonds, at specific places.

For example, some RNA molecules can cut their own nucleotide sequence, and rejoin the cut ends. This is called 'self-splicing'. What a specific RNA molecule can do depends upon other RNA molecules in the mixture. Certain RNA molecules can work together in order to make many copies of themselves, with one acting as a template, and the other as catalyst. The more successful such teams of nucleotides were, the more copies of the team members were produced. This is one of the many examples where the Universe pays a premium for cooperation.

So for life to begin, there needs to be a benign place for these basic organic molecules to interact with each other. Since Earth was at the time, very hot, and the seas were near boiling, it is unlikely that these reactions would have taken place in the very hot deep ocean, but they could have occurred in the shallows. They could have occurred deep inside Earth, and they could have taken place in mud-pools, so let's imagine that this primal activity did occur in a primordial mud-pool. Why? Because, well, I like mud! The organic molecules I referred to were amino acids, organic acids, purine, pyrimidine, nucleotides, cyanide, and so on.

Initially, they were just floating around, and randomly interacting with each other. The classical way of explaining what happened next is that at some time, totally by chance, RNA or some similar nucleic acid was formed. This was able to make copies of it. The more copies it made, the better it got at making further copies. According to this idea, the incredible complexity that we see around us is due solely to Molecular Natural Selection.

I can't accept this notion. It beggars credulity to suggest that a molecule as complex as RNA just happened by accident one fine day, or even on a cloudy one! For me, it is much more intellectually satisfying if we assume that the universe has will and creativity. For me, Natural Selection needs to be driven; otherwise, instead of a universe rich in complexity, we would just have a complex mess.

When we look at the Universe, and all the intricate things in it, it is clear to me, that it has brains, or put another way, that it is a purposeful enterprise which has as its goal the creation of life, in ever more complex forms. This is why I have used an upper case U for universe. My Universe is just as alive as we are, and this is, of course, because we are part of it. To think of the Universe as being anything other than volitional, is for me at least, an absurdity.

In order to explain this, I need to introduce the Laws of Thermodynamics. These were originally two laws, and later a third one was added. We are interested in the first two. These were at first formulated to explain the behavior of engineering systems like steam engines. The first states that the change in internal energy of a system is equal to the heat (energy) absorbed by the system, less the work done by the system on its surroundings. That is if you want to do work, you have to put in the energy; there is no such thing as a free lunch. Fair enough!

The second can be stated this way: that systems of a high level of order (organization) will tend to become disordered (disorganized) unless energy is supplied to them. An example of this is the rust on your car body, or the aging of its driver. Both are examples of nature tending to reduce an ordered system (a factory condition car or a 25-year-old healthy body at the height of its powers) to a disordered system (a pile of rust or a dead body). Unless there is investment in time and energy by the owner of the car or the body, the disorder will ensue. That is entropy!

There is evidence that we are living in an expanding Universe, whether or not this expansion is infinite is still to be determined. Because our universe is expanding, particles in it, large ones such as galaxies, and small ones are tending to run away from each other. To counteract the forces of infinite dilution of the stuff of the Universe, there are forces of attraction. Such forces are the weak and strong nuclear forces, electromagnetism, and gravity. It was these forces of order that precipitated out our galaxy, the Milky Way, from billions of particles of matter and gas in interstellar space, and then the solar system, including our lovely Earth. Luckily for us the forces of order triumphed! But where did these forces of order come from? Surely, in a naturally chaotic universe, heading towards infinite expansion, you could expect a gradual dilution of order, until, essentially nothing was left, everything being so dilute as to be not really there, but that is not what we find. We find order of almost unimaginable complexity.

Some people attribute to God the role of this organization others call it natural selection and still others believe that the Universe itself has will and wisdom.

This was the case with the invention of RNA in the first primordial mud-pool. Without self-replicating molecules, life could not have evolved. RNA and DNA, elegant and beautiful, self-replicating molecular machines were created out of the morass of organic molecules available. This set the pattern for the evolution of life. The invention of these self-replicating polynucleotides was the first major advance in the procession of life; an achievement of great subtlety that occurred in a mud-pool.

Let's now go back to our primordial mud-pool, under that same gloomy sky, and see how this happened. After a time, the pool or many pools simultaneously were filling up with self-replicating molecules. These early polynucleotides then invented genetics the computer program inside each cell. It is this programming device, which specifies whether you are a human or a virus; whether you have blue eyes, or brown; whether you will go bald early, or grow old growing hair, and whether you are likely to acquire sometime in your life, diseases such as cystic fibrosis or thalassemia.

Computer programs are made of a series of zeros or ones, which is why it is called binary code, bi from the Latin word bis which means twice or two (digits). Everything that a modern popular computer program does can be specified in code composed only of those two digits. The computer programs in your genes are based on combinations not of two digits, but of four, the four bases in DNA. Everything that a bacterium, or you, do on your own, without instruction, is spelt out in this quaternary computer code, so called because the Latin word *quartarius* means fourth part, and there is a complete copy of it in every cell of your body. The discovery of these wonderful self-replicating polynucleotides, which had the ability to act as a computer code for protein synthesis and genetics was the first major advance of the Universe.

Lots of information can be conveyed simply by the arrangement of bases in the DNA. Let me give you an example. A modern popular computer program has about one million lines of code. Now, if we assume there are about 5 bytes per line then we can conclude that this program contains 5 million bytes. We know that each byte is made up of 8 bits. Each bit is one of those zeros or ones. Therefore, such a program has about 40 million bits, if you could write this out in words, where each byte represents a letter, the computer program would fill 8 volumes of about 300 pages each. By comparison, the computer program spelt out in the base pairings in your DNA has 5 billion bits. If written out it would fill 1,000 such volumes. Each time one of your cells divide, and that can be as often as, once every 10 hours, all 1,000 volumes get transcribed from one cell to the other.

That is genetics! That is self-replication! That is what happened in the primordial mud-pool 3 or 3.5 billion years ago. Some happening! When a self-replicating polynucleotide carrying genetic information had evolved, a form of life, or something very close to life had come into existence, but it was vulnerable. It needed protection against the things that might destroy molecules, rapid changes in the physical environment. It needed a protective covering. This covering was the next major advance in the procession of life, the cell membrane.

When you wash the dishes, you probably do this with molecules of dishwashing detergent. This common household product shares properties in common with your cell membranes. The molecules in dish washing liquid are called amphiphatic molecules: they have one part that is water loving (hydrophilic), and another part that is water hating (hydrophobic). The amphiphatic detergent molecule can make grease soluble, because the hydrophobic part hates water, but loves grease. This part locks onto the animal fat, or vegetable oil, while the hydrophilic part locks onto the water in the sink. Another type of amphiphatic molecule is the phospholipid, important molecules for living things, which principally make up cell membranes.

Let's go back to our primordial mud-pool, filling with RNA. If self-replication was the most important activity defining life, the second was competition. Life succeeded in its multiplicity of forms and its extraordinary complexity because only the best suited succeeded, and went on to make further copies of themselves.

In this way the procession of life ensured not only increasing complexity, but also a type of complexity that led to organisms that were better adapted to their environment; ones that were more likely to succeed, and in life, the only measure of success is to be able to produce more copies of yourself.

We have the mud-pool is filling with RNA. What does RNA actually do? It makes proteins. Are some proteins better than others? Yes! Living things are mostly composed of proteins, more than half of the dry weight of our cells is made up of them. Therefore some proteins, better proteins, confer a competitive advantage on the organism that has them, than do inferior ones. They make the organism more likely to make copies of itself, or reproduce.

Competition, and selection through this competition, of the best qualities, or those that increase the likelihood of genetic transmission to subsequent generations, what Darwin and Wallace termed Natural Selection. But if this RNA is just free floating, making proteins from amino acids in the mud-pool, then clever RNA, that is, RNA that produces better protein, is getting no particular advantage, because the protein that it is making is just part of the common pool of protein in the primordial mud-pool.

So, sometime, in some primordial mud-pool (or in many), phospholipid molecules lined up together in a string. They tend to do this when in solution naturally. When this string of phospholipids first closed at each end around a nucleic acid core, the first biological cell had been created. The RNA inside this protected environment could now make its clever proteins, and the benefits would not be shared, but would benefit only that cell.

Greed is beautiful had reached the mud-pool. This cell, and the nucleic acids, which it contained, would have a competitive advantage over more primitive forms of biological self-replication. As we saw because it could make more copies of itself. This change, of having the RNA protected in this way, also enabled the RNA to develop itself into a new nucleic acid. We now call this new nucleic acid DNA. This is the master molecule for organizing protein synthesis, which, as we have seen, is done by instructing RNA.

RNA is a protein-making machine, and DNA can and does write the code. In this code, each triplet (three successive bases) is a code word that spells out a single amino acid. For example, GGC stands for the amino acid proline, AGA stands for the amino acid serine, and CTT stands for the amino acid glutamic acid.

The DNA code has a much more important role than merely issuing protein recipes to RNA. There are many things which we know how to do because we have been taught, such as rowing a boat or riding a bicycle, for example, but there are also things which we know how to do without ever having been taught. When, for example, was the last time someone told you how to digest an apple? Never! But you can do it. What about growing hair? When did you learn to do that? There are thousands of things which we do every day, which somehow we have always known how to do. We did not have to learn it: how to eat; how to drink; how to grow; how to digest food; how to breathe. All of these things, and many more, such as: how to make hormones, how to set tension on our vocal cords, how to make our eyes a particular color, were laid down in intricate, painstaking, and exquisite detail in our DNA code. The code, which we got from our mother and father at the time of conception; our clever system software. We have a multi-user license. There is a complete copy of this *Software of Life* in almost every one of our cells, and we don't have to pay Bill Gates a penny. Once the Universe had invented genetics, biological evolution was under way!

So, about 3 billion years ago, the first cell was formed, as we have seen, by the encircling of a nucleic acid core with a phospholipid membrane. From this time on, the evolution of life would be handled by this cell and its descendants. You and I, and all the complexity of life around us, originated from these humble and vulnerable beginnings.

Because its environment was enclosed, the cell kept whatever competitive advantage it had discovered it therefore became very successful. Originally it was simply a spherical or rod-shaped organism with a cell membrane, enclosing a single compartment (cytoplasm) containing DNA, RNA, and protein. This could be a description of a bacterium today, and some of our ancient cousins, still live in geothermal mudpools.

These cells, our first ancestors, evolved very rapidly, because they divided (reproduced) every 20 minutes. They would have used whatever nutrients were in their neighborhood.

As they became more successful, they had to colonize places different from those in which they had evolved. This caused them to change over the generations to more efficiently exploit the new environmental niche. They would then have had to invent biochemistry, so that they could more effectively utilize nutrients not always present. At this time, there was no oxygen (O_2), as only algae and photosynthetic plants, which had not evolved, produce O_2. Probably the first piece of biochemistry that the living cell developed was what we today call, anaerobic glycolysis. This is the breakdown of glucose in a way that does not require O_2. You and I still do it today. We do it for the same reason that our ancestors did, to produce energy. It was the first biological party-trick we (our ancestors actually) ever learned.

As cells became more plentiful, they began to vary, and as nutrients such as glucose came to be in short supply, certain cells came to exploit another food supply. Some of them even learned to metabolize the air itself. Two of the principal ingredients of the air at that time, were CO_2 and nitrogen. One group of cells, not in our ancestry, found a pigment called chlorophyll, which they used to make sugar from CO_2 and hydrogen sulfide (rotten-egg gas), a by-product of the frequent volcanic activity. This reaction, of making sugar from hydrogen sulfide and CO_2 produced O_2 . Later, when liquid water became more common, water was substituted for the rotten egg gas (hydrogen sulfide), and photosynthesis, as we know it today, was invented. These cells became the ancestors of all the plants in the world today, and they were also ancestors to another, simpler, life form algae. It was the algae that evolved first, and since there was an unlimited supply of these two food sources, they became very successful. Soon the world greened with photosynthetic algae, all producing a new and poisonous gas, O_2 .

O_2 a poisonous gas? Does that sound strange? It certainly to our ancestors, and many of the problems that we now meet as we age, arise because our ancestors did not evolve to live with O_2. Many of our ills reflect the uneasy compromise that they had to make with this poisonous gas, a very long time ago.

Those early cells which produced O_2 became very numerous. They also completely transformed the atmosphere, changing it from one with practically no O_2, to one with the 21 per cent O_2 seen in today's atmosphere. Furthermore, the high reactivity of O_2 made it potentially useful to organisms, since it allows them to produce much more chemical energy. Our bacteria-like ancestors and we can both do anaerobic glycolysis, as can present day bacteria. This is what happens when a piece of fruit or bread decays. But anaerobic glycolysis is an inefficient form of energy-production. When an anaerobe (a creature which can not use O_2) metabolizes glucose, it produces pyruvic acid and a small amount of energy, but when glucose is metabolized aerobically (with O_2) by another type of creature (an aerobe), it is broken down completely to CO_2 and water (H_2O) along with much more energy.

Aerobic metabolism, or respiration, produces15-times as much energy from food (glucose), than does anaerobic glycolysis.

The conditions took a turn for the worse for the anaerobes, as O_2 began to be produced in quantity by algae. To the anaerobes, including our ancestors, O_2 was poisonous. There were only four possible outcomes for them. The first was to die, and no doubt many did. Others became parasites on the aerobic cells. Some of our parasites today are in this category, and in live deep in our colon, a place with very little O_2. Others learned to live in particular environmental niches with little O_2, such as at the bottom of the sea, and in volcanoes. A fourth group were anaerobes that found a way to become aerobes. Our ancestors were in this group.

The way that our ancestors learned to use O_2 was by absorbing whole a tiny creature that made its living breaking down pyruvate by using O_2 (aerobic glycolysis). It just so happened that pyruvate was a chemical which our ancestors produced as a by-product. So these little critters probably hung around our ancestors in the beginning, trying to pick up their cast-offs, quantities of pyruvate, which, though not useful to our ancestors, was food them.

Compared with our ancestors, this little creature was an energetic little dynamo. No one knows how it first happened, but at some time this creature and our ancestor did a deal. It was a sort of marriage. They decided to live together, till death do them part. Under this deal, the creature supplied our ancestors with energy, and in exchange, our ancestors gave the creature all the pyruvate it needed. This type of arrangement, between two different creatures that results in mutual benefit, is called a symbiotic relationship, but the relationship between this formerly freewheeling dynamo and our ancestor was even more intimate.

This little creature actually started to live within our ancestors, but it never surrendered its rights as a salient creature: to possess its own

DNA, to reproduce on its own by dividing in two, and to have its own proteins. All of this happened while they lived within the substance of our ancestors. What was the name of the creature prepared to cooperate so closely with our ancestors, thereby enabling them to survive, even flourish, in a changing and very uncertain world? It was the mitochondrion. Our ancestors and this creature have been inseparable ever since, and the Universe applauded the union. Mind you, the toxicity of O_2 to our ancestors (and as a consequence to us also) did not change as a result of this union, but at least they had on board a creature that could use it, and, in return, produce heaps of energy.

The mitochondrion can be found in plant, animal and fungi cells, where it provides energy. Energy from the mitochondrion is very important, however, keeping a fire in the hearth although comfortable, is not without inherent dangers.

Flying too close to the Sun invites disaster. Our mitochondria are extremely sensitive to damage due to O_2, called oxidant damage. This tends to increase with aging, and with chronic infections. Also not only does this highly reactive element, O_2, damage the mitochondria, it can also damage other parts of the cell, such as the membrane, and this can lead to cellular death.

There could be, and I believe that there should be, a new branch of medicine, *Mitochondrial Medicine.* Indeed, we could all be attending once or twice a year, *Mitochrondrial Respiration Clinics.* There is not now such a specialty, at least not in any formal sense, and no such clinics. More is the pity! Like many of the issues in this book, mitochondrial medicine is new. It is not broadly understood, and not widely practiced. As a consequence, many aging people and those with infections are suffering oxidant stress much of which might have been prevented. They also feel chronically tired. Such *chronic fatigue* may be a symptom of poor mitochondrial function. Without mitochondria and respiration we would still be living in a geothermal mud-pool, as some of our distant cousins do today, and that is no picnic. Allowing mitochondria to specialize in energy production freed the cell membranes of our ancestors from this task.

As a result of this monumental event, these cell membranes have been able to develop ion channels, used in cell signaling. Without cellular signaling we could never have a complex nervous system. Our advanced brain and nervous system would never have developed without this union forged three billion years ago, between our ancestors and the mitochondria. What a smart move that was!

Our cells have not changed very much in two billion years. They are us, and we them. We are now a collective of cells and no longer individual unicellular organisms. We have billions of cells making up our huge brain alone. We have invented culture and an impressive civilization. Well, impressive most of the time! But everything that we are is nevertheless a consequence of our biological heritage. It does not matter if you are a Supreme Court judge or drive a cab, you, like me, share a common history ranging over these exciting of 3.5 billion years. We all can trace our ancestry to simple bacteria-like organisms that hated O_2. Many of the problems that we encounter in aging relates back to this antique heritage.

Those little critters, the mitochondria are still with us. Like diligent little furnace-men (or furnace-persons if you will), they are still doing the dangerous job of working with oxygen.

Our cells however, apart from the mitochondria, are essentially anaerobic. They evolved when the atmosphere had no oxygen, and still, oxygen is alien to them. This essential dichotomy in our nature-the fact that we are basically anaerobic, modified to live with oxygen but imperfectly, is the fundamental reason why we experience most of age-related degeneration.

CHAPTER 2

THE BUILDING BLOCKS OF THE TEMPLE: THE MOLECULES OF LIFE

Almost all aspects of life are engineered at the molecular level, and without understanding molecules we can only have a very sketchy understanding of life.

Francis Crick, British molecular biologist
What Mad Pursuit (1988)

Life as we know it is based on the carbon atom. The unique property of the carbon atom, and why it is responsible for the enormous diversity of living things that you see around you, is that this atom more than any other, is happy to form long chains. It is variety of these chains, the various ways that the atoms in them can be bound together, and the multiplicity of ways that the resulting chains can be folded, that is responsible for the complexity of living things. There are four basic types of molecules essential for the amazing variety of life around us.

These can all be joined to form long and involved chains. They are: simple sugars, which join with each other to form polysaccharides; amino acids, which join with each other to form proteins; FAs, the precursors of fats, and nucleotides, which must also be present to act as cofactors, or helpers. As well, you must of course have water. We evolved in water, and water is still essential to us, as are inorganic ions.

We will soon discuss how the carbon-based molecules, in the food we eat are converted into us through biochemistry. First though, I want to discuss energy. Energy is the power to do work. The cells of our bodies do a great deal of work. The average cell is performing thousands of biochemical reactions every minute, sometimes to supply its own needs and sometimes to make molecules for other cells, for this work it needs considerable energy.

Energy is used to do this cellular work, and other types of biological work, such as muscle contractions. Energy is also needed to drive *active transport*, the cellular mechanism that pumps molecules across a membrane against a concentration gradient. Energy is also needed to build some molecules (anabolism), and to break others down (catabolism). It is our intake of food that is the source of this energy, but we can't be expected to eat food before or immediately after every piece of biological work. If we had to do that, we would be doing nothing else.

What was needed was some way of storing energy, so that it could simply be tapped into when required. There is such a portable power supply. In fact, there are a few, but by far the most important is a compound called adenosine triphosphate (ATP).

ATP is a nucleotide, similar to the units that make up DNA and RNA. It consists of one of the bases that is in both DNA and RNA, adenine. Like the nucleotides in RNA, it also contains the sugar ribose, but unlike RNA, there is not a single phosphate bond per base, but three. These phosphate bonds, or phosphoanhydride bonds, release a large amount of energy when they are broken (hydrolyzed); around 7.3 kcal/mol. Since ATP has two of these high-energy bonds, it has two phosphate bonds that it can hydrolyze (and therefore release energy) before it reaches its low-energy state. So it may break one bond to form adenosine diphosphate (ADP), after which yet another high-energy phosphate bond is still available before it reaches its low-energy state, adenosine monophosphate.

When it reaches the latter state, it has given up all of its available energy, and like a rechargeable battery, it must then receive some energy in the form of high-energy phosphates, before it can be used for energy. These little phosphate batteries are being used, discharged, and recharged all the time. Usually an ATP molecule does not survive longer than one minute before it is used to energize some biological reaction. Even when you are at rest you would be using up 40 kg of ATP over 24 hours, but if you are exercising vigorously, then you could be using as much as 2 kg a minute. Our bodies are very busy places.

ATP provides an abundant source of instant energy for biological work, but where sustained energy production is required over a long period, say in muscle contraction, we would very soon run out of it, if we relied on ATP alone. For muscle contraction we need some other molecule, one to quickly recharge the discharged forms of ATP, AMP and adenosine diphosphate (ADP). Such a molecule does exist and is called creatine phosphate. It restores the high-energy phosphates to

ADP or AMP. In this way creatine phosphate maintains a high level of ATP, even in times of sustained muscular exertion.

You are a chemotroph! So am I. This means that we get our energy from the oxidation of food molecules, which serve as fuel. This is a form of combustion, just as a bush fire, or the internal combustion of a motor. In our bodies, however, the rate of oxidation is much, much slower. The fuel molecules that we use are glucose from CHOs, amino acids from proteins, and FAs from fats. When something is oxidized, it can be said to give up electrons. This means, for our purposes at least, oxidation. So oxidizing agents receive electrons, and the things that are oxidized, such as our food, give them up.

In creatures such as we, who breathe O_2, the oxidation of food, in its ultimate form uses the O_2 which we breathe. This is not simple combustion. It is much more controlled than that.

The way this happens is that electrons are passed from the food through a number of intermediate compounds until they are finally given to the supreme electron acceptor (oxidizing agent), O_2 itself.

These intermediate molecules are nucleotides, nicotinamide adenine dinucleotide or flavin adenine dinucleotide. Only a small part of the food we eat is oxidized, and when a molecule of glucose, which contains six carbon atoms, is used for energy production only two carbon atoms are oxidized completely, the same two every time.

These carbon atoms are in a special molecule; the star of the oxidation show! A molecule called acetyl CoA. Everything that we eat that is completely oxidized to H_2O and CO_2, whether it be from protein, carbohydrate (CHO), or fat, is first changed into this molecule before it is oxidized. Acetyl CoA is the intermediary between food and energy.

What is acetyl CoA? Discovered by Lipman in 1945, it is one of the central molecules of metabolism. Acetyl CoA is a molecule of vinegar joined to a coenzyme, or helper molecule, called coenzyme A.

Coenzymes are molecules, which do the leg-work required if metabolic reactions are to take place. They are carrier molecules: their job is usually one of taking a molecule, or part of a molecule, from one part of a reaction to another. Most of the water-soluble vitamins are components of coenzymes, including compounds such as vitamin C, a reducing agent or antioxidant, vitamin B_2 or riboflavin, a precursor of another coenzyme, FAD, and vitamin B_5 (pathothenate), a component of coenzyme A.

Let's look at what happens to each of the three principal food sources, as we convert them to energy. The primary sources of energy for the body are the CHOs. These comprise most of the organic matter on Earth, and are the main fuel of living things.

Glucose is the primary food for most of our cells, and like most other life forms we store glucose in the form of a long CHO chain. This stored form of glucose is called glycogen in humans and starch in plants. These stores are used when glucose supplies are scarce during a fast for humans and at night for plants.

Essential for life not only as energy providers, without CHOs in the form of the sugars, ribose and deoxyribose, we would not have RNA and DNA, and therefore no heredity. Without heredity there could be no life at all.

CHOs form the structural framework in the cell walls of plants and bacteria. CHOs, when linked to proteins and lipids, create a new class of compounds, glycoproteins and glycophorin, which are important for the integrity of our cell membranes. CHOs on the surface of the cell membranes enables one cell to recognize another. A sperm cell is able to bind to an egg only because it first binds to CHOs on the eggs surface. Leukocytes (white blood cells) patch up injured blood and lymphatic vessels only because adhesive proteins on their surface bind to CHOs lining the surface of the vessel.

Simple CHOs are called sugars and the simplest form of sugar is a monosaccharide. CHOs by definition are composed of carbon and water in the following scheme: $C(H_2O)n$. The most commonly known one, and the one most important in our bodies, is glucose. In this case, n=6, thus the formula for glucose is $C_6H_{12}O_6$.

This formula, however, does not tell you everything you need to know about the sugar, since sugars have a three-dimensional aspect to their chemistry. So there are a number of sugars, all with the same formula, say $C_6H_{12}O_6$, called isomers, but each representing a different sugar. These are glucose, galactose, and mannose. These three sugars differ only in the orientation of one of the OH groups with respect to the rest of the molecule. In addition, each of these sugars can have a mirror image of itself, an optical isomer, a D-form, and an L-form. The basic chemical formula of any sugar therefore, is really only the start.

Monosaccharides are so called because there is only one (*monos* is the Greek word for alone) sugar unit (saccharide). There are also larger CHOs formed when one, several, or even thousands of monosaccharide units join in a chain. A sugar formed by two simpler sugar units joining in a chain is called a disaccharide an example of which is table sugar, sucrose. A molecule formed by several sugar molecules joined together is an oligosaccharide. One formed by many sugar units joined together is called a polysaccharide (from *pollus*, which is Greek for much, and *polloi* meaning many).

Each time one sugar joins with another, a molecule of H_2O is also produced. Plant cells, like us, get energy from glucose, however unlike us, they can make their own by combining CO_2 and H_2O under the influence of sunlight. This is called photosynthesis. To do this, they use a cellular component (organelle), called a chloroplast. This organelle was probably originally a photosynthetic bacterium, which the ancestors of the algae and photosynthetic plants captured and internalized, in much the same way as the mitochondrion was acquired by our ancestors.

The chloroplast only works, when there is sunlight. If plants had not developed a way around this problem, their cells would begin to starve at night. Like us, and for much the same reason, plants have a handy glucose store, called starch. The plant breaks down this starch at night, when the chloroplast is not working, in the same way, as our glycogen is broken-down to glucose, when we are fasting.

When we eat vegetables, say, we are eating a mixture of CHOs, the most abundant of which is starch. Plants have two important polysaccharides starch the energy store and cellulose the structural polysaccharide. Cellulose is the most abundant organic material on Earth. We can't digest cellulose but a termite can. The process of digestion of sugars for us begins with the breaking down the polysaccharides (and oligosaccharides) to produce monosaccharides.

The monosaccharides are then absorbed by our gut, and ultimately delivered to the cells by the blood. Those monosaccharides, which aren't glucose are usually converted to glucose. Glucose is the principal food for most of our cells, and it is the only nutrient normally used for energy supply that can be used by the brain, retina, and the cells lining the sex glands.It is also used to supply most other cells and is the principal underlying fermentation by which yeast and bacteria can convert sugars into alcohol.

In fermentation, pyruvate the end product of anaerobic glycolysis is converted into alcohol. This does not usually happen in people unless they have yeast in their gut, which if the case, causes people to make their own alcohol, a situation called *auto-brewery syndrome.* In our metabolism, the pyruvate usually crosses over the mitochondrial membrane and takes part in a series of reactions called respiration.

Respiration is the process in the mitochondria whereby pyruvate and FAs are converted to acetyl CoA, which is then finally converted to CO_2, and H_2O. This is the final destination, not only for CHO metabolism, but also the final energy-yielding pathway for fats, and, under some conditions, proteins.

Under some conditions, the pyruvate is not taken up by the mitochondrion, but instead enters into another reaction, which in humans produces lactate. This occurs in extreme anaerobic conditions, such as when a muscle is experiencing intense activity. Lactate then builds up, and unless rest soon follows, pain called a stitch, results.

How does glucose get into our cells? Glucose levels in the blood are kept within reasonable limits by insulin, a hormone. If glucose levels in the blood are too high, then insulin is secreted by the *Islets of Langerhans* in the pancreas. This hormone causes glucose to be taken up by most cells of the body. At the level of the cell, there are specialist glucose transporters, proteins on the cell membrane, which pick up the glucose, and deliver it to the cell.

Amino acids are the basic unit of proteins. All the proteins of which we are aware are derived from only 20 amino acids. Two of which can join together to form a peptide bond, as we saw in Chapter 1. There can be many amino acids linked in long chains forming proteins. Most proteins have between 50 and 2,000 amino acids. Such a chain is a polypeptide. Proteins are made of one or more polypeptide chains.

Proteins received their name from Berzelius, who in 1838 gave them this name, derived as it was from the Greek word *proteios*, which means primary. They are the most important, versatile and useful chemicals in living cells. All life needs proteins, even viruses. Most chemical reactions in living cells are catalyzed by enzymes. Some of these enzymes increase the rate at which a chemical reaction can occur by over one million times.

All enzymes are proteins. Proteins form the structural elements of our bodies. The connective tissues, collagen and elastin, which are a types of body scaffolding, are made of them.

Proteins can transport other molecules and ions. An example of this is hemoglobin, which transports O_2 and CO_2 in the bloodstream.

Proteins are responsible for our ability to move. The contractile elements in our muscles are made of myosin and actin, both proteins. Not only are we moved by proteins, but so too are many other biological structures, even the tiny organelles inside our cells are moved on an *actin freeway*. The proteins kinesin and dynein enable single-celled animals to beat their flagella.

Proteins are used as a source of storage. Ferritin is our storage depot for iron, and casein (milk protein) is used by babies as a readily available store of amino acids.

Proteins can be messengers between cells. Insulin, the protein, which in 1955 became the first protein whose detailed sequence was worked out, is an important protein for blood-glucose regulation.

Other proteins are receptors, which communicate changed conditions to other cells. The protein rhodopsin in the retina detects light, and another protein receptor on the heart tells it to increase its rate of beating when it binds to the hormone adrenaline.

Some proteins switch genes on and off, and in some fish living near the North and South Poles, proteins that act as antifreeze compounds. Another protein in jellyfish emits a green light and another glues mussels firmly to rocks.

If there a more adaptable and versatile chemical in our bodies than a protein, I am yet to find it.

It is not just the peptide bond that makes protein chemistry so useful; mostly their versatility comes from the way the polypeptide chains are folded, their three-dimensional structure. Proteins fold in a particular way, so that the hydrophobic (water-hating) amino acid side chains are on the inside. The way that a protein is folded is determined by three bonding forces called the weak non-covalent forces, ionic bonds, and hydrogen bonds.

These bonds are so pervasive that if you denature a protein (cause it to unfold) with a chemical such as urea, and then take that chemical away, the protein will immediately resume its folded form, as though it had a memory of it.

Living systems will never run out of proteins. There are many possible forms that could be made. There are 20 amino acids so the total number of possible arrangements that could be made (say with a polypeptide of average size, about 300 amino acids long) is 20^{300}. That is a very big number! Much more than the total number of atoms in the known universe!

Proteins are also versatile. The weak non-covalent forces help a protein to fold, and to keep it in that configuration, and they also enable the protein to bind to other molecules, as they are important at binding sites. Protein polypeptide chains use binding sites to bind to other polypeptides. This enables them to assemble into much larger configurations, including sheets, filament, spheres, and helices.

Most enzymes are ball-shaped or globular proteins. Actin is a helix. Keratin, a protein in hair, horn, and nails, consists of two identical helices wound together, and collagen, the protein that gives body structures their shape, is a triple helix.

Proteins are effective because of their exceptional ability to bind to other molecules (called ligands). They are helped in this by the three-dimensional shape of the binding site, which has its particular configuration largely through the weak non-covalent bonds. Proteins also form associations with metals, such as iron and zinc, which also improves their reactivity. Protein-binding sites are specific for a particular ligand, and there are millions of them.

Consider for example, antibodies, the immune-system proteins. An antibody (or immunoglobulin) protein is a Y-shaped molecule, which has two binding sites on it. Each of which binds to a small portion on the antigen molecule. These antigen-binding sites are composed of several polypeptide loops. The antibody, when binding the antigen, folds its finger-like loops around the antigen; molecule actually lassos the antigen. This turns out to be a very efficient way of doing it, because to make the antibody specific for one antigen or another, all that the immune system has to do is to change the sequence and the length of these loops.

What happens to the proteins we eat? Proteins are degraded by digestive enzymes to form amino acids, which are taken to the liver by the portal circulation. The liver has the prime responsibility for protein metabolism. It can use these amino acids to make the proteins used by the immune system, or to make enzymes, or if glucose is in short supply, proteins can be used for making energy, by converting amino acids to metabolites themselves can be converted to glucose and oxidized in the Citric Acid Cycle.

When glucose, fats, and proteins are very scarce, as occurs in starvation, body proteins from muscles and other sources can be converted into glucose. Ketone bodies, which are often formed from this sort of reaction, as well as the conversion of fats to glucose, characteristically give the breath a sweet smell. If people are starving (or on a too strict diet), which means the same thing; their body starts to break down its own protein. They start eating themselves! These people will have on their breath the sweet smell of ketosis (high levels of ketones).

Normally, exercising muscle is spared this breakdown (catabolism), so the heart is usually not catabolized if the person is at rest, but if this starving (dieting) individual is also exercising vigorously, then the heart is only one of many exercising muscles, and it is not necessarily spared. These people may then start to live off the tissue of their own hearts and of course, this weakens it.

The third food source is fats (or lipids). It has been claimed that fats make an inordinate contribution to heart disease, and there is some truth in that, but the statement has to be heavily qualified. So let's look at the question of good fats and bad fats.

Our bodies are composed of cells. The major constituent of cell, after water, is the cell membrane. This is much more than cellular cellophane. It is a complex chemical environment, attached to which, are all manner of reactive chemicals.

Essentially composed of phospholipids (FAs attached to a phosphate ion), the cell membrane is very versatile. Sugar molecules are attached to the lipid framework of the cell membrane, to make a glycolipid. Our cells are coated with such glycolipids, as well as glycoproteins. Glycoproteins are the outcome of a union between lipid and protein and are very important for cell signaling. In fact, we are only now beginning to appreciate how important these molecules are. If your glycoproteins are disturbed, so is your whole body chemistry.

These two types of chemical personalities form the glycocalyx, which coats our cells. It is the by the glycocalyx that our cells are able to distinguish each other. The glycocalyx expresses the unique personality of each type of cell, just as our external appearance might distinguish us. At the same time, it forms a cell coat, serving as a means of protecting the cell against mechanical and chemical damage.

This phospholipid structure of the cell membrane is useful to the cell because the chemistry of lipids lends itself very well to embedded proteins, and proteins are the Merlins of cell chemistry.

The phospholipid membrane is like a chemist's bench, where the proteins perform all of their intricate magic. This is why our ancestors invented the cell membrane, when they found that they needed a chemical factory within each cell.

The membrane also makes up many of the important structures within the cell. Vital cellular structures such as the mitochondria and even the nucleus contain outer and inner membranes and our endoplasmic reticula, where many of the cellular products are made, are composed of folds of membrane.

Our cells are therefore largely composed of membranes, and the main constituents of membranes are fats (or lipids).

The most important organ we have, our brain, is also highly membranous. We are all of us fat heads. Fats are the most significant chemicals in our brains. About 200 mya, there evolved a sort of insulation around many of the important nerves. It is with us still, and called myelin.

Myelin is a membranous substance 'produced' by a cell, the Schwann cell. This insulation is achieved by the Schwann cell wrapping its own membrane round and round the nerve axon. Unlike insulation around electrical cables, the purpose is not so much to stop charge or current from leaking, but to allow it in an orderly way.

The nerve impulses jump from node to node, leaping over the myelin sheaths created by the Schwann cell. This is why our nerve impulses are sometimes called saltatory impulses (from the Latin word *saltare* meaning to jump).

This allows our nerves to transmit an impulse quickly, and it gave our ancestors an advantage over those creatures that did not have this special insulation. We would never have evolved into the advanced creatures we have become without the myelin sheath.

Our clever brain depends on the membrane, the membrane upon the phospholipids that make it up, and the phospholipids upon fatty acids (FAs). The Universe, or God if you will, has anointed us with an *oil of gladness*, just as it says in the 45th Psalm, and that oil of gladness is the composed of the fatty acids that make up the phospholipids of our cell membranes. Had we not been so anointed, we would have been very different creatures.

FAs are the basic constituents of fats. More than 100 FAs are known to occur naturally. They all have the same basic molecular structure: meaning they conform to the structure of CH_3-$(CH_2)n$-$COOH$, where the length of the hydrocarbon chain (n) can vary. In biological systems usually have an even number of carbon atoms, typically between 14 and 24. The hydrocarbon chain is almost always unbranched in the FAs found in animals.

Apart from the length of the hydrocarbon chain, there are three properties that generally make FAs different from each other.

The first is the degree to which the FA has double bonds between its carbons-the degree of saturation. The second is the location of these double bonds on the chain, and the third is whether or not the hydrogen atoms on either side of the double bond carbons are on the same side of the molecule, or are on different sides. In other words, are they cis- or trans-isomers.

What about good fats and bad fats? To put it simply, saturated fats and trans-fats (or trans-isomers) are, in general, not good for us. When a double bond is inserted between two carbons in the hydrocarbon chain, two hydrogen atoms are lost. Such a molecule is an unsaturated fatty acid, or UFA, because it is not saturated with hydrogen. A FA, which has as much hydrogen bonded as possible, is saturated with hydrogen, and is therefore a saturated fatty acid, or SaFA. Such a molecule does not have double bonds between carbons on the chain.

Since UFAs aggregate poorly, and melt at lower temperatures, they are more liquid at physiological temperatures, than saturated fatty acids (SaFAs). Thus, unsaturated fatty acids (UFAs) tend to be soft at physiological temperatures, while SaFAs tend to be hard. This is because the double bond in the UFA produces a slight local negative charge because it has a pair of extra electrons. Since like charges repel one another, UFA chains repel one another, and thereby to spread over surfaces. Thus while SaFAs tend to aggregate, UFAs tend to disperse, to move apart, to be anti-sticky. The more double bonds there are, the more they tend to disperse. These properties of UFAs help to provide the fluidity needed in cell membranes.

Fluidity allows molecules within our membranes, to swim and dive, and thereby easily perform important chemical and transport functions. UFAs with two or more double bonds are called polyunsaturated fatty acids (PUFAs). UFAs contribute to the quality of softness, so needed for healthy membranes, while SaFAs contribute to the quality of hardness. The most fluid fatty acids of all are those with the most double bonds, the PUFAs. Examples of PUFAs are oleic acid, found in olive, peanut, almond, and canola oils. Alpha-linoleic acid (LA), found in safflower, sunflower, corn, sesame, and hemp oils, and alpha-linolenic acid (LNA), found in flax, hemp, and other oils.

Oleic acid is the main FA found in olive oil. This has a double bond and therefore is a UFA, but because it only has one double bond, it is called monounsaturated. Oleic is also called nonessential, because it can be made by the body, and therefore is not essential in the diet.

Alpha-Linoleic acid is the main FA in safflower and sunflower oils. It is polyunsaturated, as it has more than one double bond. This particular polyunsaturated fatty acid (PUFA) has two, but other PUFAs can have many.

It is also said to be essential, since it can't be made by the body, and is therefore *essential in the diet.* Alpha-linolenic acid, the main FA in flax seed oil is also an essential PUFA. Because alpha-Linolenic acid (LNA) has its first double bond on the third carbon from the methyl group {the CH₃- group called the omega carbon}, reading left to right, it is called a N-3 PUFA. LA is a N-6 PUFA, because its double bond is on the sixth carbon from the omega-carbon.

A molecule of LNA is kinked because the hydrogen atoms either side of the double bonds are on the same side of the molecule. In such a position they repel each other, and the carbon chain kinks on the side opposite the hydrogens, to take up space away from the repelling H atoms. Such a kinked molecule is called a cis-fatty acid (c-FA), while the opposite, where the hydrogen atoms are on opposite sides of the double bond, is called trans-FAs (t-FA). t-Fas are not kinked, lie flat against each other, and so tend to be solid at low temperatures.

Cis- is the favored form (isomer) in nature. So if you substitute t-FAs for the c-FAs, many of the biological enzymes in our membrane structures do not recognize them. These FAs therefore become useless for structural purposes, and can only be used as fuel. c-FAs on the other hand, are treated preciously and tend to be used for the important business of cell membrane building, and prostaglandin (important local hormones, which we will discuss later) synthesis, as well as for fuel.

Our enzymes use t-FAs and c-FAs differently. Fatty acids are converted into ketone bodies (acetoacetate and 3-hydroxybutyrate), which can be used by the mitochondria to make energy, but the rate of production of ketone bodies from t-FAs is slower than the rate at which they are produced from c-FAs. It is for this reason that a diet high in t-FAs can be a problem for the heart.

The main source of fuel for our hearts is the FA, and if the breakdown of t-FAs is slower than the breakdown of c-FAs, this could mean that such a diet is likely to lower the performance of the heart, and this could have important, even fatal, consequences.

When t-FAs are incorporated into cell membranes their permeability is detrimentally affected. It is tantamount to punching holes in the cells, and molecules normally kept out of a cell are thereby able to get inside. A diet high in t-FAs injures cells, diminishes cell vitality, and immune function.

Further, an intake of t-FAs worsens an existing essential FA deficiency, by interfering with the enzyme systems that turn FAs into the UFA-derivatives highly prized by the body. These enzymes are especially concentrated in the brain, retina, adrenals, and testes.

t-FAs interfere also with the production of prostaglandins (PGs), or local hormones that regulate many important biological functions, such as muscle tone in the wall of the arteries, regulate platelet stickiness, regulate kidney function, the inflammatory response, and immune competence. t-FAs and saturated FAs should be avoided if possible, but the eating of all fats is certainly not to be avoided.

Fats are necessary for health. Our cell membranes, and our brains, are mostly composed of them. They form covalent bonds with proteins, and this helps to target the protein to the correct part of the cell membrane. They are a source of stored energy.

They are important in the production of hormones, and other intracellular messengers. They are also responsible for the integrity cell membrane, the retina of our eyes, and of the brain.

What we call *fat* on our bodies (technically depot fat or adipose tissue) is a concentrated form of stored energy. It is made up of triacylglycerols (or triglycerides), and is something which we have put away for a rainy day, a famine actually. Of course in Western countries now, famines are few and far between, so it usually just sits there. The places where we store fat are under genetic control, and tend to be, to some degree at least, idiosyncratic. Fat tends to be deposited in different places in men and women. Men tend to put on fat around their abdomen, while pre-menopausal women tend to put on fat on their bottoms, breasts, and hips.

In 1949 Eugene Kennedy and Albert Lehninger were the first to demonstrate that FAs, like pyruvate (from glucose), are oxidized in the mitochondria. The complete oxidation of one FA, say palmitate, produces 106 ATP molecules, whereas the complete oxidation of a pyruvate molecule in glucose metabolism produces only 15 ATP molecules. The complete oxidation of glucose, which results in two pyruvate molecules, yields 30 ATP molecules. This is a much less energetic reaction than the oxidation of a FA, which yields more than 3-times as much energy.

Whatever is the source of the ATP, glucose or FAs, the oxidation in mitochondria is enormously efficient, giving an efficiency of about 50 percent. The average car engine can only manage around 20 to 30 percent.

Let's now look at the mitochondrion, that friend of our ancestors, without which we would still be in the primordial mud-pool. The mitochondrion consists of an outer membrane that surrounds an inner matrix. This inner matrix is highly concentrated mixture of hundreds of enzymes. The enzymes used in the Citric Acid Cycle, for the oxidation of pyruvate and FAs, live in the outer part of the mitochondrion, the matrix. Deeper inside still is an inner membrane. This inner membrane is folded into folds, or cristae, so the surface area is greatly increased. The inner membrane contains the enzymes for making ATP and some transport enzymes in the respiratory chain.

Deep within the mitochondrion, at the inner membrane, electrons are carried by two high-energy carriers, through a complex of enzymes, and finally given to elemental O_2 the same O_2 , which we breathe. O_2 is the ultimate oxidizer. The process by which electrons are passed down this electron chain is called *oxidative phosphorylation,* and its purpose is to produce ATP, the portable energy molecule. Without O_2 at the end of the electron chain, as the final electron acceptor (oxidizer), we would not be able to make ATP, and therefore not able to supply energy to biological processes.

This reaction, oxidative phosphorylation, is the great gift that the mitochondria gave our ancestors. It provides most of our energy, but it is a two-edged sword, because it also produces *free radicals*, which as well shall see, are an important cause of disease.

Everything that you do requires energy supplied by the high-energy phosphate bonds in ATP. When you exercise at the gym, you are using ATP. When you think and remember your brain is using ATP. When your muscle cells make proteins, you are using ATP. The energy that your heart uses to pump is supplied by ATP. When the cells in the testes need energy to make sperm, they use ATP, and when those same sperm set out on their marathon swim of confluence with the egg, their beating tails are powered by ATP. ATP is what runs us, and the principal supplier of ATP is the mitochondrion, through oxidative phosphorylation.

If a molecule is capable of being oxidized, it can give electrons. Whatever molecule receives these electrons is the oxidizing agent. When a molecule of glucose is oxidized by glycolysis, it produces two molecules of pyruvate, 2 molecules of ATP, and two molecules of NADH. The production of two molecules of pyruvate from one molecule of glucose occurs in virtually every cell. This reaction does not require O_2 and produces only a small amount of ATP (2 molecules which represents only 3 percent of the available energy). This was the limit on energy production experienced by our ancient ancestors before they acquired mitochondria.

To get a really large amount of ATP, you need to completely oxidize the pyruvate to CO_2 and H_2O. This occurs only in the Citric Acid Cycle, in the mitochondrion.

The formula for the oxidation of pyruvate is:
$$C_3H_4O_3 + 22O_2 \text{ produces } 3CO_2 + 2H_2O$$

This actually represents two processes, the first is the oxidation of pyruvate to CO_2 and H in the citric acid cycle:
$$C_3H_4O_3 + 3H_2O \text{ produces } 3CO_2 + 10H.$$

The H in these reactions represents two electrons.

The second process is the conversion of the 10H to form one molecule of ATP:
$$10H + 22O_2 \text{ produces } 5H_2O + 14 \text{ ATP}$$

The electrons are carried by reduced electron carriers, such as NAD^+ and FAD. When they are carrying the electrons, they take the form NADH and $FADH_2$. Remember that donating an electron is the same as oxidation and that the molecule donating the electron is being oxidized. So in oxidative phosphorylation since electrons are passed down a chain, it is a chain of oxidation.

It is in this way, that electrons derived from the oxidation of food molecules are transferred along a series of electron carriers called the electron transport chain. Each time the electron is transferred, energy is released, and this energy is used to pump a proton across the membrane. When this happens, an electrochemical gradient is formed. Such an ionic gradient across a membrane is a form of energy storage like the charging of a battery. This energy can be used to do work and the work that is done when the protons flow back in the opposite direction is driving the conversion of ADP into ATP.

This is the complex process, discovered in a mud-pool 3 billion years ago, by which, the food we eat is turned into energy. Electron transfer from the chain drives protons in one direction, and their subsequent flow back drives the phosphorylation of ADP to ATP.

This reaction can also be driven in the other direction, causing the hydrolysis of ATP, if energy is needed. The only problem left to deal with is what to do with the electrons at the end of the transport chain. Each time the electrons are passed some energy is lost, so you need something at the end of the chain, which is a superb electron acceptor, or oxidizing agent, and what could that be? Oxygen itself, of course.

Have you noticed that as you age you seem to have less energy? Most of the energy produced by biological systems is from respiration. Perhaps if we are suffering from an energy shortage, the electron transport chain of respiration is the place to look for answers.

There are three respiratory enzyme complexes in the inner mitochrondrial membrane, and there are two electron carriers, ubiquinone or Coenzyme Q_{10} and cytochrome c. If these electron carriers are not working, respiration is sluggish, and ultimately, we end up with a (personal) energy crisis.

The proton pump on the inner mitochondrial membrane is like a turbine, which drives the creation of high-energy phosphates, ATP and ADP. It is ATP that is the highest energy source. The enzyme that does this is ATP synthase. This ancient enzyme was the one that our anaerobic ancestors coveted, when they saw those little mitochondria floating around to mud-pool quietly turning pyruvate and FAs into stacks of ATP, and having energy to burn. It is present in the mitochondria of animal cells, the chloroplasts of plants and algae, and in the cell membranes of bacteria.

Coenzyme Q_{10}, one of the mitochondrial electron carriers, is an amazing compound. Dr Karl Folkers, one of the pioneers of using this natural substance therapeutically has stated that once our levels of Coenzyme Q_{10} drop by 75 percent of an expected norm, we will die. He also maintains that a fall of only 25 percent will result in disease.

All plants and animal cells contain Coenzyme Q_{10}, so it is available in everything we eat that is why it is called ubiquinone, since it is ubiquitous. Some foods however, rapidly respiring ones, like beef heart, are particularly rich in it. But if you are not partial to eating heart, a good steak, or any other skeletal muscle also contains a good supply of Coenzyme Q_{10}.

Coenzyme Q_{10} can be made by our bodies, and therefore it probably does not qualify to be called a vitamin, which is something that is essential for life and which *can't* be made by the body. The body's synthesis of Coenzyme Q_{10} requires the vitamins, B_6, C, B_{12}, B_2, folic acid, niacin, and pantothenic acid as coenzymes. So although technically it is not a vitamin itself, it can only be made with them.

There are as the name suggests, ten Coenzyme Qs, but only Q_{10} is of the most common form occurring in man. Coenzyme Q_{10} belongs to the chemical family of quinines, it is a quinone derivative, and is of the group of natural substances, which give to the vegetables and fruit in which they are found, color, fragrance and astringency. The color of tomatoes and carrots come from two such compounds, lycopene and beta-carotene respectively. These are polyphenols, very important for health, as we shall see later, and they are chemically, cousins of Coenzyme Q_{10}. All of these compounds are also potent antioxidants.

Mitochondria are not static little spheres. They literally go to the areas where they are needed for energy supply. In the heart muscle for example, mitochondria wrap themselves around the contracting filaments of heart muscle, so that these tissues have a constant supply of ATP. In a similar way they wrap themselves around the tail of the sperm to supply it with energy for its long, difficult and dangerous journey.

Many of the diseases of aging are ischemic, ones in which the blood, oxygen and nutritional supply to an important organ like the heart is restricted or blocked. This ischemia may be because respiration itself has broken down, as in tissues with abnormal mitochondria, or it may be ischemia with a more obvious cause, such as atherosclerosis. Whatever the cause, people suffering ischemic disease should benefit from therapy with Coenzyme Q_{10}.

Our mitochondria are susceptible to damage, and this damage is cumulative, and manifests more in aging. In my view, the taking of Coenzyme Q_{10} either in a food source or as a supplement, can be efficacious in most aging people, because most of us, with aging, have some form of respiratory (mitochondrial) dysfunction.

For sometime now Coenzyme Q_{10} and its relatives have been found to be useful as an immune-system stimulant; as an adjunct in the treatment of ischemic heart, liver and brain disease; as a protector in various forms of cell damage; to assist in recovery from reperfusion injury; as a powerful antioxidant; in the management of myocardial failure; in the treatment of cardiomyopathy, as well as of congestive heart failure, and even of periodontitis. It has been used with success to improve cardiac output after valve-replacement surgery, and also in other forms of low cardiac output and hypertension.

Coenzyme Q_{10} is not only for ischemic diseases and cancer, but may be used to provide more energy to an aging body, in circumstances where inefficient cellular respiration is the cause of the energy loss.

Given that it is so potentially useful, do GPs prescribe it? Not usually! Do we see articles about this wonderful and cheap therapy? Not many! Maybe that is the problem, it is too cheap, and we like medication that is expensive. Certainly, the pharmaceutical companies do. I think it about time we took faulty respiration and this wonderful and inexpensive therapy more seriously.

CHAPTER 3

CONSUMED BY A SLOW FIRE

Tarnished with rust,
She that was young and fair
Fallen to dust
Oscar Wilde, *Requiescat, 1881*

As we enter in the 21st century, we enter a world that will be very different than any world that has ever existed before. There are certain sociological changes, which are going on now, the like of which have not occurred since the end of the 18th century when people first moved from family farms to factories. Today, as the three technologies of computers, television and telephone converge, the world is becoming connected in a way that has never been available before.

What will matter in the 21st century is information. Those who have access to it will do well, and conversely those on the other side of the *digital divide* will not. We can expect to see much strife in the 21st century because of these inequalities, the beginnings of which we can see around us already.

The potential for pain that the present holds is not being aided by the behavior of some of the world's great corporations, as they pursue profits through globalization.

Globalization is not a bad thing per se. Indeed, as this convergence of the communication technologies proceeds it is inevitable. The world for example, could only benefit from a global perspective on the environment, on poverty, or on the education of women, which is the only sure way of limiting global population. Such initiatives, if they ever proceeded contain within them the seeds of global harmony and well-being.

What is being passed-off as Globalism today contains only the seeds of adversity. It is the pursuit of profits by global corporations, without due concern for the communities that they serve, combined with an inability or unwillingness of Governments to tame the economic system, and thereby make it more user-friendly.

This fiduciary failure, grandly styled Globalization, is creating inequality and marginalizing very large numbers of people, perhaps forever, and such a situation can only result in social strife. One can see the beginnings of this social disorder occurring now, and it will only increase as time goes by.

Governments need to act, because the corporations will not do it on their own. They are merely entities designed to return profits to their shareholders. They have no ethics outside of that, and in the main they are run by fearful, greedy and unimaginative men.

It is true, that some of these behemouths are in a sense, more powerful than any single national government, but many world governments, acting globally, could bring them to heel. Of course, this presupposes politicians with the V-thing; you know, Vision

Considering the current batch of world leaders, one can't help feeling that they will avoid such imaginative and courageous action until forced to do something; the V-thing being in short supply. When it does occur however, as it must eventually, it will be True Globalism. Globalism for the benefit of the many, not the few.

There is another way in which the 21st century will be unique, it will be the *Century of the Aged*. A declining birth rate in many countries compounded with the extraordinary increase in life expectancy, which occurred throughout much of the 20th century, means that in the 21st century there will be a very large proportion of old people in most countries.

The numbers of elderly people (those aged between 45 and 65) has been increasing since the early part of the 20th century, and by the year 2005, the worldwide numbers of this group is expected to reach 410 million, from 290 million twenty years earlier.

Does this mean that all these old people have to be a burden on society? Does being old necessarily mean being sick and dependent on others? In order to answer that question, we must first pose another: what is aging?

Aging is a progressive loss of function, which seems to be inevitable. The sad truth is that as we progress through adulthood towards old age most of our physiological functions gradually decline.

Our senses decline in their ability to tell us about the world outside, as we suffer from presbyacusis (old man's hearing) and senile cataracts in the eyes. We get dental and periodontal problems.

We may have difficulties swallowing. We tend to get overweight, as a consequence of which we could end up with hiatus hernia. Our obesity as we age can also produce a form of diabetes. Whether or not we acquire diabetes, we will very likely have a reduced capacity to deal with sugar. Intestinal absorption, pancreatic and liver function, all tend to decline. We can lose gut flora, which may contribute to the tendency in old age for our serum cholesterol levels to rise.

We may suffer from diverticulosis, as the mechanical properties of our gut tend to decline. Our stomach becomes no longer so good at making HCl. We may experience a deficiency of vitamin B^{12} , and perhaps suffer from pernicious anemia. The lining of our stomach may decline in health, leading to gastritis, and perhaps gastric cancer. We may become susceptible to Helicobacter pylori (H. pylori) infection, which may lead to duodenal ulcers or gastric cancer. We may develop colonic cancer.

The capacity of our bodies for cellular protein synthesis declines. We tend to lose muscle tone, and our muscles no longer respond, as we would want them to do. There is a loss of muscle mass and strength, an increase in fat mass, and a decrease in bone density.

Our lungs tend to shrink, and become stiffer. Our BP will rise. Our arteries will become harder, very likely resulting in hypertension, coronary heart disease, and stroke. The chances of us getting cancer are much higher as we age. At the same time, our libido will decline. Men may suffer from impotence, and women will experience what is perhaps the most dramatic health-related event of aging, menopause.

What is menopause? Menopause (meaning the cessation of menses, or menstrual bleeding) is a relatively sudden, near total collapse of the ovaries, which occurs in most women around the age of 50 (or 51 in most developed countries) years. The ovaries, which had throughout the woman's reproductive life produced estrogen and progesterone, are suddenly unable to do so. This is not the end of the woman's estrogen production. The post-menopausal ovary still produces small quantities for about another decade. As well, the ovary produces testosterone (male sex hormone), a hormone also produced by the women's adrenal glands. The adrenal glands, which sit like caps on the kidneys, continue to produce testosterone, as they had before menopause.

Testosterone in a woman is responsible for the growth of pubic and underarm hair, and libido. Although the adrenal gland produces some testosterone in the woman's body, most of her supply of this hormone comes from her ovaries.

In the woman's peripheral tissues, such as fat, brain, liver, and breast cells, some female testosterone is post-menopausally converted to estrogen but compared with the pre-menopausal levels the amount of estrogen produced in this way is small. Women who have more fat will convert more estrogen, and will therefore have more circulating estrogen than lean post-menopausal women.

This sudden and remarkable change seems to be based on two events. One occurs in the ovaries themselves. Women have only a limited number of eggs. Before a female child is born, in mid-term of her mother's pregnancy, she has seven million potential eggs. When the girl is born, the number of eggs has decreased to one million. By the time she reaches puberty, she has 40,000, and around the age of 50, she is usually down to very few or none, thus triggering menopause. There is some individual variation in the exact year at which this occurs, but for most women, it is well on its way by 50.

It is not a matter of them all having been released by the ovary (ovulation), many simply die. The eggs are produced in an ovarian follicle, and it is these egg follicles that produce most of the estrogen, and all of the progesterone. When the ovary runs out of eggs it also runs out of follicles, and therefore the hormones that they produce.

This is one cause of menopause. The other is in the brain. It is the hypothalamus that is the part of the brain that is in direct contact with the master gland of the body, the pituitary gland. It seems that there is a pacemaker, or a timekeeper, in this hypothalamic-pituitary relationship. At around 50 years, the hypothalamus, says: *That's it, we don't need to stimulate ovulation any more! She is now too old to have healthy babies! When this order is given, the pituitary gland simply switches the ovaries off.*

Why do women have to undergo menopause? Probably for the better raising of children. Human beings have very large, highly developed brains. It is the secret of their evolutionary success. The human brain is so highly developed that babies must be born before the brain is finished its development. If gestation lasted longer, the baby's head would never fit through the mother's pelvic girdle.

As a consequence of the fact that their brains are still relatively *unfinished*, human babies are very vulnerable, when born and immediately thereafter, compared with the newborns of other species. As a consequence a large amount of time and resources must be spent in the education and care of the youngster. This may require the help, not only of both parents, but their parents as well, the child's grandparents.

If the grandmother was still able to have children of her own, these would compete for her attention. So it is quite probable that evolution has seen to it that the *Grannies* are available to help with their children's child-raising. This might be accomplished by switching off the functional capacity of the ovary, as happens, in menopause. It is notable that the only other mammal, which undergoes a sharp and dramatic menopause, the Pilot Whale, is also a creature, where the parent's parents have a role in child-raising.

Menopause is often accompanied by depressed mood, an increase in the risk of cardiovascular disease, a loss of bone mass (osteoporosis), dryness of skin and vagina, bladder problems, aches and pains, alterations to sleep patterns, and a change in the muscle tone of arterioles of the skin, resulting in hot flashes. Hot flashes are caused because the hypothalamus has as one of its functions the regulation of temperature. When you are too hot, it causes arterioles near the skin of open up, causing more blood to flow to the skin. When this happens, body temperature falls, as heat is exchanged between the blood and the environment outside.

The particular part of the hypothalamus responsible for temperature regulation in this way is dependent for its efficient activity on estrogen. At menopause, when it suddenly senses a sharp decline in estrogen, it goes a little crazy, acting as though the woman is hot, when she is not, and therefore sending blood to the skin.

Men go through a similar thing an age-related reproductive-hormone decline, but it is nowhere near as dramatic or as sudden as with women. It has been called *andropause*, and is slower and much more gradual.

During aging, there is a gradual decline is testosterone levels in males, caused by a decrease in the numbers of, and the secretory capacity of, hormone-secreting cells in the testes. This too seems to be under the same hypothalamic-pituitary control as with women.

In men, the age-related decline in testosterone may be accompanied by a tendency towards osteoporosis, a loss of libido, a loss of sexual potency, and perhaps some of their masculinity. Old men and women are much more alike than are young men and women.

The ability of our bodies to respond to changes in temperature will decline, as we get older. Our brains could well decline in many cognitive (thinking) functions, especially memory. There will be a decline in immune function as we age, which results in a progressive inability to ward off infectious illness, so that if we live long enough most of us will ultimately die of pneumonia, the old man's friend.

Aging is, to a large extent, written into our DNA, our system software. That this aging will involve some loss of function is something we can't avoid. Whether or not we become sick, incapacitated, and/or dependent, depends on the degree to which we suffer from the chronic degenerative diseases of aging. These are conditions such as osteoporosis, diabetes, arthritis (osteoarthritis, gout, and rheumatoid arthritis), diabetes, coronary heart disease, high BP, dementia, digestive illnesses such as gallstones and cancer. The extent to which we suffer from many of these diseases is, at least to some extent, under our own control.

The chronic degenerative diseases of aging are certainly more prevalent now ever. But they are not inventions of the 20th century, or even the 21st. Our species has suffered from them for a very long time- some of the pre-Homo early human ancestors certainly did. Evidence of human remains from France dating to 40,000 years ago, called the Old Man of La'Chapelle aux Saints shows that he suffered from osteoarthritis. In Egyptian mummies, we see evidence of gallstones, as well as osteoarthritis and atherosclerosis. In many early cultures, including Asian, Greek, and Egyptian, we have unmistakable evidence of hypertension, as well as insulin dependent diabetes mellitus (IDDM) and non-insulin dependent diabetes mellitus (NIDDM).

There are identifiable environment causes for these diseases. For example, they are for the most part, ailments of affluence, and although it is mostly in this century that affluence has existed in large parts of the world, the trend to affluence has been underway throughout the last two centuries, and there are reports of diseases like coronary heart disease, atherosclerosis, and NIDDM, amongst the rich throughout this period. Indeed, the association of diabetes and gout to obesity was reported as early as the Greek and Roman times, during the Middle Ages and thereafter.

By contrast other degenerative diseases well known today, such as hypertension, coronary heart disease (CHD), cerebrovascular disease (stroke), cancer, and the neurological disorders of Parkinson's (PD) and Alzheimer's diseases (AD), were not reported until the 19th and early 20th centuries.

Of course, chronic degenerative diseases of old age were not common in former times, because few people actually reached old age. Most died in their 40s and 50s usually from infectious diseases. It was only during the last century when life expectancies have improved quite markedly however, that we have the privilege of suffering from the diseases of old age, en masse. These diseases typically affect people over 40 years, and that was a very small percent age of the population, even in Europe only 300 years ago. Also of course, the fact that they were rare in previous eras means that they received little attention.

In order to understand these diseases, it may be instructive to look at what has changed, between these earlier societies and our own modern cosmopolitan one. Our populations have a much larger proportion over the age of 50 years. Our children mature earlier in today's metropolitan societies, starting at age 11 to 12 for girls. This compares with around 16 in earlier societies, or even modern rural and isolated ones. So although children now reach an earlier reproductive maturation, being physiologically ready for childbearing at about 13 to 14 years, and have a longer reproductive period than earlier societies, they have their first pregnancy later in life.

This trend has existed since the 19th century, and also distinguishes modern cosmopolitan societies from modern rural societies. In most ancient societies and in modern hunter-gather ones, a woman tends to be pregnant or lactating continuously from puberty to menopause.

Throughout most of human evolution, women had high levels of progesterone and lactating hormones, compared with their levels of estrogen. The reverse characterizes women of modern metropolitan societies because of an earlier sexual maturation, later and fewer pregnancies, and a longer reproductive period. This change in hormone profiles of modern women is an important factor contributing to the significantly higher levels of breast and cervical cancer.

This is far from the only mortality and morbidity risk factor associated with modern living. In this modern metropolitan world we have substituted fatty foods for fiber-dense foods, increased our exposure to pollutants, stress, and radiation. For most of our evolutionary history we were animals who, on the whole, consumed fiber-rich foods, and had to exercise to provide for our needs. Today, we eat a predominance of fat- and sugar-rich foods, and exercise little. These changes alone contribute greatly to cardiovascular disease, cancer, diabetes, osteoporosis, irritable bowel syndrome, hypertension, and obesity.

We are also today, subjected to a bewildering array of toxic substances, many of which were unknown throughout the greater part of human evolution. Some tend to suppress our immune systems and overload our livers, leading to a propensity for allergies, and for chronic infections.

Our low-fiber and high-fat diet has contributed to such diseases as diverticulosis and colorectal cancer. The high levels of vascular diseases and NIDDM today are also largely traceable to this diet, which compounded with lack of physical exercise, leads to obesity and high levels of blood lipids.

Not only the quantity, but also the type of fats consumed by modern people and their livestock has changed over the last 100 years. The importance of this in relation to the higher incidence of the degenerative diseases of aging can't be overstated.

Modern people eat and feed their animals more processed food than did previous populations. This has had the effect of converting many of their essential FAs into long-chain saturated ones, and in a proportionately larger amount of trans-isomers.

Why have these changes in diet been so fatal to us? The reason for this lies in our evolutionary history. Throughout most of their evolutionary history, our ancestors were vegetarians, with a fancy for the odd insect. Meat-eating could not have started in any real sense, until *Australopithecus Aferensis* (*A. Aferensis*), one of the early humans, learned to walk upright, and that was a mere 3.5 million years ago (mya).

The only early human, which we know for sure, was a meat-eater was Homo *habilis* (*H. habilis*) only 2 mya. We know this because this creature left behind tools used for butchering large animals. But whether it was 3.5 or 2 mya is beside the point; in evolutionary terms, it was yesterday.

Even after our ancestors had learned to eat other large animals, this would not have been something they did every day. A large animal, like a woolly mammoth, is hard to capture and kill. Most large animals are stronger than humans, and often faster. They also have had a long evolutionary history; time enough to have learned some good defenses against such predation.

The big advantage that humans had was their big brain. This meant they could build sophisticated weapons and traps, and most importantly, hunt in cooperative groups. Even so, capturing a large animal was a big job, and for most of our evolutionary history, fatty meat was a luxury. A compact and highly concentrated form of energy like fatty food was prized.

A supply of fatty food could keep a tribe going for a lot longer than the roots and leaves of plants. So we were designed by our evolution to value it. This is why it tastes so good! That is evolution's way of putting a value on it.

This is also why it is that you see so much fatty food in the supermarket today, mostly in various forms of manufactured (processed) foods. The processed foods in the supermarket today often have an inordinate amount of fat because the companies that make these foods know that people prefer fatty foods. So do many companies, which supply mass-produced food to the market.

Today though, we do not have to wait for someone to kill a bull (or even a woolly mammoth) to get a good supply of fatty food. It is available anywhere, and our bodies, which evolved treating fat as a seldomly acquired treat, do not know how to deal with it in the amounts in which it is found in the modern Western diet.

This idea, first put by J.V. Neal in 1962, maintains that fat is something put away for a rainy day. Today though, fatty food is now the norm in affluent human populations, for the first time in 350,000 generations.

Our diet and lifestyle, characterized by plenty, is a significant factor in making us sick in old age. CHD, vascular disease, obesity, NIDDM, and even cancer to some extent are diseases of an affluent society. They are also diseases of old age.

The fat story is still more complicated than that. It is not so much that our diet is high in fat that leads to these diseases, but more that it is high in the wrong types of fat. Inuit populations in Greenland and Alaska have a very high intake of fat. Usually more than 40 percent of their calories are represented by fat. But they do not suffer from these chronic degenerative diseases, as do Americans and Western Europeans.

If you compare the ratio of deaths from coronary heart disease (CHD) between Intuit people and Danes, the Danes die about twice as much from CHD. Why? Because the Danes who consume about as much fat as the Intuit, have twice as much *saturated fat.*

The Intuit diet is different in another respect: most of the fat they eat comes from cold-water marine animals and fish, which are high in N-3 PUFAs. This type of FA seems to be protective against CHD. Indeed, when Intuit people leave Greenland to live in Denmark, they develop the same blood-lipid concentrations as the Danes, and, one presumes, will develop similar diseases.

The protection against CHD that the Intuit enjoyed arose because in order for fat to lead to CHD it needs to be changed to low-density lipoprotein (LDL) by the liver. Saturated fat from terrestrial sources readily undergoes this transformation with N-3 FAs from marine animals less so.

Another way in which our diet today is unusual, in historical terms, is that salt is now plentiful. Ancient man had to go to a lot of trouble to take salt from seawater or to mine it. Salt was so prized in Roman times it was often used to pay the army, and this is the origin of the modern word salary.

Certain people and groups have been found to be sensitive to salt. It was found by the Intersalt studies that the tendency of BP to rise with age was related to the intake of salt. This occurred whether or not the people taking the salt had been previously diagnosed with hypertension. However, salt does not affect everyone equally in this regard. For example, African Americans are more sensitive than Americans of European or British descent.

This difference in people no doubt has an evolutionary explanation, for example, it may be that Africans coming from a hot climate had to conserve salt lost in sweat during the day and, salt was treated more preciously by their physiology, compared with that of people from the colder Europe. Superimposed over all this are free radicals, which contribute in substantially to many of these degenerative diseases.

Free radicals are not restricted to the present time, but in earlier eras and societies humans tended to eat more fruit and vegetables than today. This had the effect of bolstering our natural antioxidant defenses. A high fat diet itself leads to the generation of free radicals, because the sugars and fats in it themselves become potent sources of oxidation.

Is there any good news? Yes! A progressive degeneration into helplessness, sickness, and dependency is not necessarily the inevitable future for us all. Being sick is not inevitable because we now have a good idea of what aspects of behavior and diet may cause the illnesses of aging. Many of the worst aspects of these chronic degenerative diseases of aging are, at least, intensified, if not caused, by the effects of free radicals and other oxidant chemicals. Collectively this type of injury is referred to as oxidant stress.

When this is compounded with a tendency to eat too much, to take too little exercise, to eat the wrong type of fats and too few protective vegetables, we have a good picture of why it is, that aging and illness so often go together.

Let me put forward an appealing, romantic but perhaps totally implausible scenario. Our ancestors, those anaerobic, bacteria-like creatures living in the thermal mud-pools wished to be conscious-beings.

The Universe granted this wish, but first they had to make a Faustian bargain. They had to acquire those fiery furnaces, the mitochondria. There was no other way.

For most of our lives, our mitochondria are good and faithful servants, but as we age, the fallout from these quadrillions of fiery furnaces takes its toll, and, ultimately, as Karen Reiser, a well known researcher in the area, so aptly put it, *oxidative phosphorylation becomes the slow fire that consumes us.*

If you want to understand what free radicals are, look around! Rust is an example; here free radicals are rapidly converting a formerly impressive iron structure to iron oxide dust.

Free radicals are highly reactive agents associated with O_2, that have an unpaired electron. Electrons like to be in paired orbitals, and free radicals are desperate to get a partner for their unpaired electron. This makes them promiscuous in what they react with.

These wanton free radicals contribute to many of the unwelcome changes accompany aging by reacting with body structures in an attempt to find an electron. This type of reaction, of a free radical reacting with a body structure and changing it chemically, is called oxidant stress, and oxidant stress is the principal cause of age-related degeneration.

Why do we call it *oxidant* stress? We saw before that the giving of an electron is equivalent to oxidation, where the molecule donating the electron is being oxidized, and that receiving it is the oxidizing agent. Free radicals can pair their lone electron by taking an electron from some other chemical in the body, a sugar or a fat. In doing so they are oxidizing it, and such damage is therefore called oxidant stress, while the chemicals that stop this process, such as vitamin C, vitamin E, and beta-carotene are called antioxidants.

Not all oxidants however are free radicals. Some chemicals such as hydrogen peroxide (H_2O_2) also have the power to oxidize and yet are not radicals. It is for this reason that this whole class of oxidant biological molecules has been called *Radical Oxygen Species (ROS)*.

The maximum lifespan of an animal is directly related to the level of its natural defense against oxidant damage. Humans have the longest maximum life span of any mammal, and consume more energy over this lifespan on a per weight basis. They also have the best defense of any mammal against oxidant damage, but even so, ultimately oxidant damage ultimately leads to their demise. Its does this by resulting in what we describe as the degenerative diseases of aging.

Free radicals are constantly produced in many of our metabolic reactions. The reactions of the respiratory chain in the mitochondria are an important source. Phagocytes and monocytes in our immune system, which have harnessed respiratory free radicals as weapons to kill microbes, obviously produce many.

Free radicals are also produced in the synthesis of prostaglandins. Those hormone-like substances are generated from UFAs in cell membranes. They are very useful chemicals, which have many actions, including the constriction and dilation of arteries, the stimulation of pain-nerve endings, and the promotion and inhibition of blood clotting, to name only a few.

Free radicals are also produced by the cytochrome *P-450* system in the liver-one of the detoxification pathways.

Free radicals vary in their degree of reactivity, and therefore in how dangerous they are. The hydroxyl radicals are the most dangerous. They react with almost all the molecules in living cells. Wherever hydroxyl radicals are formed, they damage the cellular structures next to them.

Free radicals can be produced by radiation, such as UV light. Ionizing radiation causes the fission of hydrogen and oxygen bond in water, releasing harmful hydroxyl radicals. This is why exposure to too much UV light is dangerous; ionizing radiation, by producing hydroxyl radicals, can disrupt proteins, lipids (in cell membranes), and even the precious genetic material, the DNA in the cell nucleus. Sometimes resulting in a melanoma.

The cells that line arteries, vascular endothelial cells, phagocytes, some brain cells and others all produce another free radical, nitric oxide. This radical is made from a common amino acid, L-arginine. Nitric oxide is much less harmful than the hydroxyl radical and may even have some beneficial qualities-it dilates blood vessels; it may be a neurotransmitter (a messenger chemical between nerve cells), and is used by macrophages to kill parasites.

A free radical closely related to oxygen is the superoxide ion. Many phagocytic cells, neutrophils, monocytes, macrophages and eosinophils, to kill bacteria and viruses, produce this radical. The superoxide ion may even by produced by cells such as fibroblasts, and lymphocytes, as part of their cell-signaling apparatus.

Cell signaling involves the sending of special chemicals between cells which are received by particular receptors on the surface membrane of the receiving cell. It is by this means that cells talk to each other. This system of cellular communication is vital for many reasons, including the regulation of (tissue) growth.

Reperfusion is the situation whereby an organ, say the heart, which has been ischemic for some time, suddenly gets a good supply of blood, perhaps after by-pass surgery. This sudden availability of oxygenated blood causes the cells that line the arteries of the heart (endothelial cells) to produce the superoxide ion, which in turn, causes injury, known as reperfusion injury. We are not sure whether the endothelial cells produce the superoxide ion all the time, or only after an insult like a reperfusion injury.

Free radicals such as the superoxide ion are not just produced to kill bacteria, or made by the body. They are produced in the body by cytochrome-based reactions.

Cytochromes (the word is derived from Greek words meaning cell colors) are colored pigments that do an electron hot-potato act like the electron chain in the mitochondria. Certain chemicals in the body, such as tetrahydrofolates, catecholamines, and reduced flavins, produce superoxide ions when they react with O_2. This is called autoxidation. Metal ions, such as iron and copper, might be important for these autoxidation reactions.

Some of the electrons entering the respiratory ETC of the mitochondria leak out of the reaction, and result in the production of superoxide ions. About one to three percent is a good estimate for the leakage of electrons available from all sources, and much of this goes into the formation of superoxide ions. Humans therefore, could produce something like 1.72 kg of superoxide ions per year when at rest, and 17 kg per year during muscular exertion. That is quite a lot of this dangerous chemical.

What do superoxide ions do in the body? They can react with vital enzymes, such as NADH dehydrogenase, in the respiration ETC, and inactivate them. Superoxide ions also inactivate nitric oxide by reacting with it. Nitric oxide has a role of dilating (or relaxing arteries), so when superoxide inactivates it, it causes a constriction of arteries, which might be an important contributor to hypertension, or high BP. Superoxide ions are also involved in atherosclerosis. When superoxide ions do react with nitric oxide they produce another ROS called peroxynitrite, as well as the hydroxyl radical. Peroxynitrite can oxidize the sulfydryl groups (-SH) on proteins, rendering them biologically altered; it can also be converted to two other products, nitrogen dioxide, and the nitronium ion. Nitrogen dioxide is active in the oxidation of lipids and the nitronium ion alters important proteins, such as phenylalanine and tyrosine.

Free ions of iron and copper are powerful catalysts to oxidation in our bodies. Most of the time these ions are bound to proteins, such as ferritin, where they do no harm, but hydrogen peroxide and the superoxide ion can cause them to be removed from this safe storage, where they become very dangerous indeed, and contribute greatly to the oxidation of our lipids. It is for this reason that hydrogen peroxide and the superoxide ion must be removed as soon as they are formed to prevent this release of metal ions, called the Fenton reaction.

Free radicals and oxidant stress contribute greatly to tissue damage and disease. Whatever cellular structure a free radical is near often loses an electron. Such a structure is usually one with a large number of electrons, such as: the cell membrane, a membrane around an organelle such as a mitochondrion, a protein, or a sugar.

Such a reaction completely alters the structure's biological activity and this may be a vital role, like that of a protein on a membrane receptor. If the molecule that the free radical disturbs is a sugar, this often results in the production of further oxidant molecules. Free radicals can get electrons from DNA, where they disrupt the production of proteins, and even our genetic code itself.

Certain otherwise inexplicable changes, which occur as we age, are associated with the failure of cell membrane receptors. For example, although we may be making sufficient insulin, our cells often fail to react to it. Similarly, with aging the receptors that govern the rate at which our hearts beat tend to sometimes fail to respond to their hormone. Why is it that aging often seems to cause our cellular receptors to fail in this way? A common denominator that connects the failure of membrane receptors and aging might be the disruption caused to these delicate structures receptors by oxidant stress.

This damage could occur in a number of ways. Free radicals may react directly with the receptor-proteins and alter them chemically. Or other oxidant species related to glucose in our blood, Advanced Glycation End Products (AGEs), may cause the proteins in many of our cell membrane receptors to become cross-linked, and so render them biologically useless.

The free radicals generated by the cell in the mitochondria, over time destroy them or make them abnormal. This means that with age we have less available energy, since it is our mitochondria that generate our energy, and they have become abnormal. Furthermore, our receptors are driven by energy (ATP), so, in time, as the cellular energy levels (ATP) fall lower as a result of faulty mitochondrial function, these receptors cease to function.

This affects, not only receptors for hormones, but also the sodium/potassium ATPase (Na^+/K^+ ATPase) pumps used for active transport in the cell, and the calcium pumps, used for cellular signaling. We have known since 1947 of the importance of calcium pumps on the cell membrane. The evidence is already there that certain ROS, such as hydrogen peroxide disrupt these calcium pumps, and they keep the cell viable by pumping out calcium. If these calcium pumps fail, because they lack energy, or are otherwise disrupted by ROS, then the balance of calcium within the cell (calcium homeostasis) is upset, and the cell can die, or become abnormal. Oxidant stress therefore, may be the principle cause of such abnormal cellular functioning.

Not all ROS are produced within our bodies, some are introduced from outside. Such chemicals, which are foreign to the body but have been introduced into the body's environment, are called xenobiotics. Two seriously oxidant xenobiotics are benzene and ozone.

Benzene is an ubiquitous pollutant of the today. It is produced by jet engines and sprayed on cities as they fly over. Benzene and its metabolites generate hydrogen peroxide, the hydroxyl radical and the superoxide ion, as well as $1O_2$. These are known to damage chromosomes of the blood and bone marrow, places where benzene and its metabolites tend to accumulate. Benzene is a component of fuels, especially aviation fuel, and gets sprayed over cities by jet aircraft.

Motor-vehicle emissions contain many pollutants including nitrogen monoxide, which is converted into nitrogen dioxide, which catalyzes the formation of ozone. Ozone itself an oxidant, also contributes to asthma, and there have been many reports from all over the world, of associations between proximity to traffic and wheezing, particularly among children. This is something that town planners should keep in mind. Take my hometown, Sydney, Australia. The outer western suburbs of Sydney have among the highest incidence of childhood asthma in the world. This is largely due to the fact that Sydney forms a large basin, bound by the Tasman Sea on the east and the Blue Mountains on the west. Most afternoons, onshore winds move most of the vehicular air pollution from the city to the outer west, where the mountains stop its progress. As a consequence, the children in these suburbs experience a high incidence of asthma. Similar circumstances exist in many of the world's great cities.

Research supports a close association between pollution with respiratory disorders, such as asthma. Outdoor pollutants including ozone, sulfur dioxide, sulfuric acid, and oxides of nitrogen cause broncho-constriction in susceptible individuals and these are all components of the photochemical smog prevalent is many industrialized cities today

The most common xenobiotic is cigarette smoke. A cigarette is a device for administering an addictive drug, like a syringe. Nicotine causes free radical formation and the peroxidation of lipids, but the cigarette is more dangerous than the nicotine. Two researchers, Church and Pryor, have shown that each puff of a cigarette has 10^{14} free radicals in the gas, and 10^{15} in the tar phase. That is more than one million times the number of people on the earth, and you get that number of free radicals with every puff! It is not surprising then that smokers have lower levels of antioxidants such as vitamin C, selenium, and vitamin E than nonsmokers, that smoking markedly increases the risk of myocardial infarction in men and women, as well as also increasing the chances of acquiring lung, cervical, and bladder cancer.

Our ancestors developed a protein called actin about 3 billion years ago, and used it to make a cytoskeleton-a sort of rapid-transport system, by which cellular products are moved around the cell. ROS can inter-act with blood sugars causing cross-linking of the proteins of the cytoskeleton. This causes the cytoskeleton to become abnormal. Things can't move around the cell easily, and the cell's normal biological func-tion is disturbed.

Cells exposed to ROS experience an energy (ATP) shortage because the normal functioning of the mitochondria has been upset. Why is the mitochondrion so badly affected by oxidant stress? Because it is com-posed of membranes! It is circumscribed by a membrane, and it has an inner membrane at its core. The latter membrane is where the actual energy producing reaction (oxidative phosphorylation) takes place.

Membranes are particularly susceptible to oxidant stress and this is why surface receptor proteins and the mitochondria are so badly affect-ed. Why? Because membranes are composed mostly of lipids, and ROS like hydrogen peroxide react with these lipids to produce lipid hydroperoxides. The reaction is catalyzed by transition metals such as iron and copper, and these are usually freely available only in an oxidant environment.

Perhaps the most serious injury that oxidant stress can do is to dam-age the DNA. This is because if damage is done to say, a cell membrane, then the worst that can happen is that the cell will die, and provided that it is not heart or brain it will be replaced. But when you damage DNA, the genetic material, it is possible that this damage gets trans-mitted through all of that cell's progeny.

Cellular DNA is damaged, in many cell types, only minutes after exposure to oxidants. Hydroxyl radicals generated from water and H_2O_2 is particularly dangerous in initiating this type of damage. H_2O_2 is made by neutrophils, it is one of the weapons they use against microbes, and it has the capacity to be changed to hydroxyl radicals when in the pres-ence of ferrous (iron) ions (Fe^{2+}).

Iron is the most abundant metal in Earth's crust, and there is a lot of iron in our bodies. Most of this is locked away in storage, bound to two proteins, hemoglobin and ferritin. Under some conditions of oxidant stress, Fe^{2+} is released, and catalyzes some of these oxidant reactions.

The damage caused by the hydroxyl radicals is manifested by breaks in the DNA strand. DNA does have repair systems, but after consistent oxidant injury of this type, they become overloaded. The gradual accumulation of damaged DNA, and its transmission across generations of cells, is the main reason why the incidence of cancers increases with age.

So we are left with the following cascade of events. Some cellular damage inflicted by infection, mechanical or thermal shock, toxic agents, or allergy, causes an inflammatory response. As a result of this, leukocytes produce H_2O_2, which penetrates the cell to reach important structures within the cell, particularly the cell membranes, and protein-based membrane receptors. Damage to the mitochondria, those highly membranous and therefore vulnerable organelles, affects everything in the cell that uses energy.

The mitochondria are particularly susceptible to oxidant damage because the reaction, which they harbor, respiration, itself generates free radicals, and a small percent age of these respiratory free radicals leak out of the ETC to do damage elsewhere, especially superoxide ions.

Nearly everything that the cell is capable of doing depends on energy from the mitochondria. This includes the sodium-potassium pumps that drive membrane transport, and the calcium channels which regulate cell signaling, both vital for the survival of the cell.

H_2O_2 is converted to hydroxyl radicals, which then causes damage to nuclear DNA. In addition, inflammatory processes, which can be started off by oxidant damage, draw in phagocytic cells, which add to the oxidant burden. As mitochondria are damaged, cellular energy drops. As the cytoskeleton is damaged, normal biological function becomes impossible. As the DNA is damaged, the chances of cellular abnormalities and ultimately cancer increase.

Although oxidant stress is common, the disastrous consequences are not so readily observable, not immediately anyway!

The cell first adopts certain fail-safe practices: the antioxidant defenses and DNA repair systems, but even these are not always sufficient to keep up extensive and recurring damage. Under such circumstances the cell often becomes abnormal.

Antioxidant defenses have evolved in living organisms, to remove superoxide ions and hydrogen peroxide. The three enzyme systems, superoxide dismutase (SOD), catalase (CAT), and glutathione peroxidase (GPX), are the basis of the body's antioxidant defense system. In addition to these, there are other natural defenses: antioxidants. These are a number of molecules and protein fragments found in the body that harmlessly react with and eliminate free radicals (free radical scavengers) and other ROS. These include bilirubin, a by-product of red cell recycling, and glutathione, a tripeptide formed from the combination of three amino acids, glycine, glutamic acid, and cysteine.

Glutathione is found in various foods, including asparagus, avocados and watermelon, and is known to be particularly important to good health. Glutathione levels are highest in the healthiest old people. Another important substance is uric acid, which can scavenge free radicals, but also can remove iron ions (Fe^{2+}), which if left free in the body would be added to the oxidant load.

SOD removes superoxide ions by converting them to H_2O_2. H_2O_2 is dangerous, so there are two enzyme dedicated to its removal. One, catalase (CAT), is usually located near the SOD to remove its product, and the other is the selenoprotein glutathione peroxidase (GPX). This enzyme has the metal selenium at its active site. GPX removes H_2O_2 by using peroxide's oxidizing potential to oxidize reduced glutathione (GSH) forming the oxidized glutathione (GSSG). The reduced form of glutathione is later regenerated, by means of another enzyme glutathione reductase. GPX can remove the oxidized forms of FAs, called fatty acid peroxides by converting them to alcohols.

As well as these natural antioxidant enzymes, there are other molecules in our food that also scavenge ROS. These are the antioxidant vitamins. The best known of which are alpha-tocopherol (vitamin E), beta-carotene, and ascorbic acid (vitamin C). Beta-carotene is a member of a large family of antioxidants, the carotenes. There are very many carotenes. They, along with their relative vitamin A, are part of a larger group called the retinols. Indeed, beta-carotene is a metabolic precursor of vitamin A, and is sometimes called provitamin A. Vitamin E, vitamin A, and the carotenes are hydrophobic, which means they tend to like a fatty (lipid) environment. Vitamin C is hydrophilic or water loving rather than fat loving (hydrophobic).

Vitamin E is the most important antioxidant in lipid (fat) mediums, such as those in the membranes of cells and mitochondria. In this environment hydroxyl radicals is the most dangerous radical.

What makes vitamin E so useful is that it can intercept a free radical and render it harmless. When an hydroxyl radical makes an attack on the PUFAs in a membrane, it interacts with molecular oxygen to produce a lipid peroxyl radical, which in turn gives rise to a lipid hydroperoxide. Vitamin E works as an antioxidant by transferring a hydrogen atom from its phenolic ring to form a tocopheroxyl radical.

The tocopheroxyl radical inactivates the hydroxyl radical rendering it biologically harmless by stringing two such radicals together to form a non-radical. Vitamin E is then regenerated from the tocopheroxyl radical by a system that involves vitamin C. Therefore, vitamin E and vitamin C are both required to control membrane damage initiated by free radicals. Vitamin E works in the membrane, arresting the radical by sacrificing itself to the radical, and vitamin C regenerates the peroxidized vitamin E. Ubiquinol (reduced coenzyme Q_{10}) may also act as a recycler of vitamin E. One molecule of vitamin E can protect 1,000 lipid molecules.

Why are lipid peroxides so disruptive to membranes? Because lipids (in membranes) are uncharged or hydrophobic. However, when a lipid peroxide is formed, a charged or hydrophilic element is added. The amphiphatic lipid hydroperoxide has a part that wants to stay in the membrane and another which wants to leave it. The result of this tug-of-war, as with most wars, is destruction.

As well as by the intervention by vitamin E, lipid hydroperoxides can be purged from the membrane by glutathione. There is in the membrane an enzyme called phospholipase A^2. If this enzyme is activated by the presence of the lipid ydroperoxide, the peroxidized-FA will be reduced to a harmless hydroxy acid. This reaction requires the catalytic assistance of GPX. Because GPX is dependent on the metal selenium, the dietary adequacy of this metal is important.

If the lipid hydroperoxide is not removed by one of these two means, it may undergo further oxidant reactions catalyzed by Fe^{2+} producing yet more ROS. So that not only does it do damage itself, but it starts a chain reaction of radicals that continue the destruction.

Vitamin C is a good antioxidant against several reactive oxygen species. It scavenges the hydroxyl radicals and superoxide ions radicals, hypochlorous acid, ozone, and H_2O_2. It also removes $1O_2$ in solution, prevents the breakdown of heme, and inhibits lipid peroxidation. Foods that are high in vitamin C are green leafy vegetables and fruit. The same foods that are protective against heart disease and cancer.

Vitamin A is essential for many biological processes. It is often made in the body from precursors called provitamins, such as beta-carotene and others. These provitamin carotenoids are found in fruit and vegetables. All of the carotenoids and vitamin A (the retinols) are antioxidants. Vitamin A deficiency is linked with dryness of the eyes and thickening of the conjunctiva (xerophthalmia), particularly among undernourished children.

Because free radicals are generated by respiration and other cytochrome-based reactions, we make them when we are respiring the most-when exercising vigorously. Exercise will increase oxidant stress because our mitochondria are working harder, and therefore there is a greater chance of leakage of free radicals and electrons from the mitochondrial ETC. Also, exercising muscles may produce transient ischemia, as the muscle works so hard it temporarily overwhelms the capacity of the circulation to supply it. If this exercise consists of heavy exertion, which is not followed by rest, there is a build-up of lactic acid, causing a stitch, and then additional oxidant damage caused by reperfusion of the ischemic muscle, and consequent production of the superoxide ions. Finally, when lactic acid builds up, as it will in anaerobic exercise, it may reduce levels of those important electron carriers involved in respiration, NADH and NADPH. This may compromise antioxidant function.

Strenuous exercise does result in the increased production of free radicals, and the subsequent oxidation of lipids and proteins. But usually, this is counterbalanced by the antioxidant defense system, including vitamin C, uric acid, and vitamin E that has developed over our long evolutionary history to protect exercising muscles.

In rapidly respiring tissues, such as exercising muscles, it is clear that most of the damage that is likely to occur is going to be in the mitochondrial membranes. Vitamin E is the antioxidant that lives and works in the phospholipid bilayer that makes up cell and mitochondrial membranes, and so will be most effective against lipid peroxidation caused by exercise. In several studies vitamin E supplementation has caused a reduction in the damage caused by lipid peroxidation after exercise. Of course, vitamin C would also be needed because it regenerates vitamin E.

Does this mean that we should not exercise? No! Exercise is very beneficial, but when we do have vigorous exercise, our need for vitamins E and C is greater.

Many people (including me) will be very pleased to hear that red wine is high in flavonols, and these antioxidant properties may contribute to a perceived reduced risk of CHD in red wine drinkers, the so-called *French Paradox*. It is thought that the flavonols in red wine inhibit the oxidation of blood lipids that is a leading cause of atherosclerois. Chocolate, you may also be pleased to hear, is also a rich source of polyphenols as well; lipids are resistant to oxidation for two hours after eating chocolate. In the interest of balance, it must also be added, that chocolate also contains some saturated fat, which is not good, but then on the other hand, the fats in chocolate are much less dangerous than those in meat. Chocolate is also a very rich source of magnesium, a very important mineral. So the occasional night of chocolate and wine (pink champagne?) may not be such a bad idea.

Many studies have shown that a diet rich in fruit and vegetables is protective against cancer. It is probably the polyphenols that are responsible for this.

A good source of polyphenols is tea. Tea-leaves contain more than 35 percent of their dry weight as polyphenols, but their antioxidant potential is affected by manufacturing processes.

Green tea is richest in flavonols. In black tea, most of the polyphenols (catechins) have been oxidized to thearubigens and theaflavins, which give the tea its distinctive red-brown color. The fermentation of green tea produces black tea, and this reaction causes the simple polyphenols in the green tea to form those complex compounds of condensation. Green tea has something like five-times the amount of polyphenols. The polyphenols in tea can also react with, and be inactivated by, casein proteins in milk. So, drink your tea without milk, and if you do so, remember that green tea is better than black.

A very important event in the development of ill health and in the degenerative diseases of aging is membrane damage due to lipid oxidation (or peroxidation). There are approximately one billion lipid molecules in the plasma membrane of a small animal cell. When a membrane is healthy, the cell it envelopes is also healthy. Conversely, when a membrane is not healthy, the cell becomes diseased. What makes membranes healthy? Fluidity!

All living things need to be soft and fluid to be healthy. When they become hardened they are on the road to death. When the membrane loses its fluidity, it begins to lose its functions. What are the factors that make a cell membrane lose its fluidity? The first is temperature, as membranes get close to freezing point they tend to crystallize. This is not an issue for most of us. The second is FA constitution, and that does affect us. The third factor that alters the fluidity of cell membranes is lipid peroxidation.

As our cell membranes age, they become stiffer, and less fluid. This occurs because of two processes that usually occur together the increasing saturation of the membrane lipids, and an increase in their peroxidation. Age-related membrane hardening has a devastating effect on the membrane. A number of membrane transport processes and enzyme activities can be shown to cease, when the bilayer viscosity (membrane hardness) is experimentally increased beyond a threshold level.

Let's look at the processes involved in this increase in membrane viscosity. Firstly, the constitution of the lipids that make up the membrane changes with aging. PUFAs of the omega-6 (N-6) and omega-3 (N-3) type decrease steadily, and saturated fats tend to increase. These changes relate directly to the types of fats we eat.

SaFA molecules incorporated into our membranes from our diet do not have double bonds to give the molecules kinks, thereby stopping them coalescing together. Instead they pack densely, and tend therefore to be solid at low temperatures.

Saturated fats therefore, are hard fats, and too many saturated fats in our diet, and therefore in our membranes, contribute markedly to the hardening of membranes that occurs with aging.

Cell membranes are made from sheets of phospholipids, interspersed and separated by a molecule of cholesterol. Unlike the phospholipid molecules, the cholesterol is not soft and malleable.

It is a hard nuggetty molecule, made from tightly constructed sterol rings. This molecule sits between the phospholipid sheets like reinforcing girders in a concrete building. The cholesterol, though a stiff and non-deforming molecule, is necessary because it gives strength in the membrane, and tends to keep the phospholipid sheets separated, preventing them from coalescing into a soft fatty mass.

The cholesterol molecules also make the membrane less permeable to small molecules and water. For these reasons some cholesterol is necessary but too much of it is not good. We need the rigid cholesterol molecule between the sheets-phospholipid sheets that is!

This is why, a completely fat-free diet may cause more harm than good, especially to the brain, which is mostly made of cell membranes (white matter). But too much of it, makes the whole membrane take on the stiff and unyielding quality of the cholesterol, and produces hard cell membranes. There is a direct correlation between membrane microviscosity (hardness), and the ratio of cholesterol/ phospholipids in the serum. Since plasma lipids can penetrate cell membranes readily, high cholesterol in the plasma is reflected in membrane composition. The level of cholesterol in the membrane needs to be within strict parameters for the membrane to work at optimal capacity. Very small changes in the cholesterol level are enough to completely disturb membrane functions.

Increased cholesterol is common in aging and we can expect that the fluidity of membranes be decreased under this cholesterol enrichment. As serum cholesterol rises, and the ratio of cholesterol to phospholipids also rises, the membranes become stiffer. Indeed, this may be why lymphocyte activation seems to fail with aging.

Lipids in our cells also tend to be oxidized as we age. The free-radical oxidation of membrane lipids is part of a chain reaction. In this way, a single hit of a free radical can initiate a series of reactions that can cause the oxidation of many molecules. These free-radical membrane interactions affect the chemical and physical properties of the membrane. The FAs that help to make up the membrane are changed from the "good" cis- double-bond type, to the "bad" trans-form by lipid peroxidation.

As lipid peroxidation in membranes proceeds, the membranes become more rigid. Both the phospholipids and the membrane proteins are attacked by free radicals.

Many cells are killed by free radicals where there are not antioxidants to soak them up, and so prevent the damage. One cell hat has been studied in this way is the red blood cell (erythrocyte). These cells are particularly susceptible to oxidation because their membranes are rich in PUFAs, which can be readily oxidized, and they are continuously exposed to oxygen As an erythrocyte becomes mortally oxidized it gradually spills or leaks out some of its important constituents: first the potassium ions leak out, followed by calcium ions, then lactate dehydrogenase, aspartate tranaminase, Hb, and the cell dies.

The quality of hardness in cell membranes is the basis of the degeneration that occurs with aging. This membrane hardening is exacerbated by: the replacement of cis-fatty acids with trans-fatty acids; the replacement of UFAs acids with saturated ones; and the greatly increased levels of hard cholesterol molecules between the phospholipid sheets. To finish the cell off completely, there is one final insult: the lipid peroxidation tends to turn healthy cis- double-bonded FAs into unhealthy trans-double bonded FAs. This alters the membrane proteins, and causes the membrane to develop pores instigating a breakdown of the ionic pumps, and resulting in the loss of cell integrity. The cell becomes a darkened hulk; its spark of life extinguished, it slowly extrudes its vital stuff to the interstitial medium, and simply ceases to exist entirely.

Let me set up for you a series of events that I think is likely to happen when we experience a significant source of oxidant damage, say exposure to ionizing radiation. This could be UV light from exposure to the sun, r other forms of radiation, such as X-ray. As the radiation hits the skin, and penetrates to the cell membranes, some of the lipids in the cell membranes are oxidized.

Peroxidized lipids themselves give off free radicals and spread the oxidation even further, but they are at first prevented from initiating this chain reaction by the cholesterol lying in the cell membranes between the phospholipid sheets. As the level of radiation becomes too much for the cholesterol-buffer to manage, a chain-reaction of oxidized lipid radicals begins. Lipid-generated free radicals are formed from the oxidation products themselves, as well as hydroxyl radical formed from the fission of cellular water.

If you are lucky, you will have some vitamin E, beta-carotene, or ubiquinol in your cell membrane, which will neutralize (quench) the free radicals. If not, the cellular damage will be high, perhaps fatally so. H_2O_2 will be generated from hydroxyl radicals, and cellular damage begins to occur within minutes of exposure to these ROS. If this damage is extensive, the cell will issue an alarm call. This alarm call will attract the body's phagocytes to the site, and these in turn will start blasting away at neighboring cells with H_2O_2, as a full blown inflammatory response ensues. Inflammation is the body's reaction to injury, and inflammation and free-radical damage go hand in hand. Because of the many free radicals in the area, and the previous free-radical damage, some of the iron normally locked up safely in ferritin, is released as free Fe^{2+}. This catalyzes encourages the conversion of the H_2O_2 to hydroxyl radicals, the most dangerous of all.

It can then be speculated, that if such an oxidant cascade occurs near muscle or other tissues where insulin receptors are found in high numbers, such membrane damage may cause an alteration in that receptor. As these reactions occur repeatedly, more and more of the insulin-receptor proteins may be damaged, and it may then become difficult for the body to regulate blood-glucose. The pancreas will release insulin when the glucose levels rise, but the cells that normally respond to the insulin, such as the fat and muscle cells, will fail to respond, and this results in a high level of blood-glucose most of the time. The glucose reacts with some proteins, specifically lysine and hydroxylysine, to produce AGEs, such as carboxymethylhydroxylysine (CML). Thirty percent of the original lysine groups present on a protein are incorporated into CML after glycation. The Fe^{2+}catalyzed oxidation of membrane FAs in the presence of protein, which is ubiquitous on cell membranes, is enough to create CML. Indeed, the peroxidation of lipids can be the main source of AGEs, such as CML.

Some of the macrophages recognize the AGEs as trouble, and begin to consume them, but their generation has become so widespread that the macrophages can't keep up with it. The AGEs in this oxidant and glucose-enriched environment bring about the reaction between glucose and amino acids in the cytoskeleton proteins. As a consequence, this cellular super-highway ceases to function properly, and the cell goes into terminal decline. AGEs react, not only with the cytoskeleton's actin protein, but also with the proteins that make up collagen that is the basic structural material of living organisms, the scaffolding that holds everything else together.

The accumulation of glycated proteins on collagen affects the mechanical and chemical properties of collagen, and the behavior of the cells that rest on the collagen membrane. Cells on a membrane of glycated collagen begin to act strangely, in terms of growth, differentiation, motility, gene expression, and response to cytokines. For example, the adhesion and spreading of endothelial cells are decreased when those cells are on a basement membrane that contains glycated collagen and laminin. Under these circumstances, if you have an injury to an artery, and anyone with lipid peroxidation will have some damage to arteries, then the endothelium, or the damaged lining of the artery, is less able to restore it to a normal condition.

The relationship between glycation and aging is very close! The relationship between aging and non-enzymatic glycation has been studied for more than 20 years. We have all noticed how it is that with aging our skin becomes less elastic. One group measured these age-associated changes in skin elasticity in subjects aged 20-85, and compared it to the measurements of AGEs in those subjects. What they saw was not only did persons between those two ages show a marked decline in skin elasticity, but they also had a fivefold increase in AGEs over the period.

Another group conducting a similar experiment, which studied the amount of glycation of skin collagen in subjects aged 42 to 78, said that the increase in glycation was exponential. It is glycation of skin collagen that makes our skin get thinner and less elastic. So if you are looking for something to blame for the changes in your appearance as you age, look no further than oxidant stress and protein glycation.

Let us now look at the damage that may be brought to the nucleus of the cell by free radicals. Nuclei, deep within cell, are not immune to oxidant attack by free radicals. Cells, especially heavily respiring cells, contain a large number of mitochondria. The liver alone, has between 2000 to 2500 mitochondria in the average cell. Altogether, each of us carries 20 quadrillion (thousand trillion) mitochondria.

Mitochondria, which work with O_2 all the time, are very susceptible to oxidant damage themselves, and are a major source of free radicals, which attack other structures near them. In 1971, Briton Chance, from Philadelphia, first established that mitochondria produced H_2O_2 as a byproduct of respiration, and seven years later Nohl and Hegner described the fact that aging mitochondria tended to increase in levels of superoxide radicals and H_2O_2. It was this paper, more than 20 years ago, that first proposed that an age-related stimulation of mitochondrial oxygen activation was responsible for an imbalance between pro-oxidants and antioxidants.

DNA is a highly complex molecule, and susceptible to oxidation. There are products from the oxidation of DNA that can be measured. These markers of oxidation consist of 5-hydroxymethyluracil, 8-hydroxy 2'-deoxyguanosine, and 8-hydroxy 2'-deoxyguanosine. It has been estimated that the levels of 8-hydroxy 2'-deoxyguanosine are 16-times higher in mitochondrial DNA than in nuclear DNA. This corresponds to a damage rate of 1 in every 8 000 bases.

This extraordinarily high rate of damage is due to the fact that mitochondrial DNA is very close to respiration-generated ROS, and normally mitochondria are not well equipped with antioxidants. Animals that have a high metabolic rate and a short life span, such as rats, excrete about 15 times more 5-hydroxymethyluracil per kilogram of body weight than do humans. The high exposure of mitochondrial DNA to oxidant damage of course has absolutely everything to do with the failure of the mitochondria as we age.

Of the ROS that we have discussed, neither superoxide nor H_2O_2, can, on their own, cause damage to the DNA in the nuclei of our cells. These ROS are only dangerous to DNA because they undergo a reaction catalyzed by the transition metals, iron and copper, to form hydroxyl radicals. Free-radical-induced damage to nuclear DNA occurs from hydroxyl radicals and lipid peroxides. Ionizing radiation is not merely a superficial phenomenon. Such radiation can be absorbed directly by the DNA of our cells, causing the breakdown of its bases, or as we saw, by the generation of hydroxyl radicals from H_2O near the nucleus. It is the hydroxyl radicals, which are responsible for most of the damage done to DNA.

Superoxide ions cause the release of Fe^{2+} from its safe storage in ferritin, and make it available to catalyze the conversion of H_2O_2 to hydroxyl radicals. In addition, Fe^{2+} can be released from heme protein damaged by H_2O_2, and the heme protein is ubiquitous, being found in mitochondria, red cells and muscle.

Metals such as iron are bound to proteins associated with DNA, so such a Fenton reaction is probably very common in the nucleus. All you need to release the iron from its protein-bound form is some superoxide ions.

H_2O_2 is also common in our diet, being present in tea, coffee, edible oil, and even in tap water, as well as being formed in the atmosphere photochemically from polluted fog droplets.

H_2O_2 can also be found in cigarette smoke, with man-made mineral fibers, such as rock wool, glass wool, and silicate fibers, and even more dangerous ones such as asbestos. Silicates such as asbestos can cause fibrosis of the lung and lung cancer when inhaled, and they also contain some iron that can feed into the Fenton reaction.

The combination of asbestos inhalation with smoking results in a large increase (50 to 90 times) in lung cancer. This compares with an increase of only 5 to 10-times the risk with one factor alone. This suggests a synergistic increase in the breaking of DNA chains when asbestos and cigarette smoke are combined. It is also fairly clear that this reaction must involve hydroxyl radicals.

Cigarette smoking is one-stop shop, supplying everything needed for DNA damage with the iron (from asbestos), silicates and asbestos, and H_2O_2; it is all there When you combine that with additional carcinogens in cigarette smoke, such as benzo[a]pyrene, and hydroquinone, you got it all in one neat package, available at all supermarkets and corner stores.

Once formed by whatever means, hydroxyl radicals remove hydrogen atoms from the sugar deoxyribose, and forms double bonds in some of the DNA bases. Damage through reaction of hydroxyl radicals with the DNA bases is the most common form of destruction. The totality of these reactions is to cause a DNA strand to break. There are two types of breaks possible: a single strand break (SSB), which is a break to only one of the strands in the DNA double helix, and a double strand break (DSB), a break to both stands. An SSB is serious but does not usually cause the death of the cell. DSBs are more serious. They usually result in permanent damage to the genetic material, and sometimes in cell death. DSBs are usually caused by a large amount of radiation energy being deposited in one place, resulting in multiple hydroxyl radical attacks on the DNA double-strand. It is multiple, not single, attacks by hydroxyl radicals that are responsible for DSBs.

When DNA sustains damage to its bases it can cause the misdirection of DNA polymerases, the molecules that build a new DNA molecule from the old one. They are responsible for DNA replication. The misdirection of the polymerase molecule will cause the incorporation of the wrong base opposite the damaged base during replication of the DNA. This is the first step towards the initiation of cancer.

Lipid peroxides are the products created when any lipid undergoes oxidation, from free radicals or any other cause. They themselves are able to break DNA strands. The peroxidation of lipids increases with age, very likely because of the continued exposure to free radicals and other oxidants, compounded by the decline in antioxidant defenses that also occurs with aging. It is very likely that the damage rendered to nuclear DNA by lipid peroxides is not from the peroxide itself, which is unlikely to reach nuclear DNA, but by other products of lipid peroxidation, possibly the carbonyl products. These are small enough to diffuse into the region of the DNA, and are possible mutagens (agents which cause cells to change their behavior).

Like weary veteran gladiators, as we get older we accumulate damage. Largely oxidant processes combined with protein glycation cause this. Age spots occur on our skin and inside as well. The accumulation of an aging pigment, lipofuscin, occurs in many organs, including the cells of the liver and brain. Lipid peroxides cause lipofuscin, and the reaction may be accelerated by the availability of free Fe^{2+} ions. Such markers as age-spots are just the outward expression of the extensive oxidation that occurs with aging in the secret rooms of our bodies.

The aging rate is proportional to metabolic rate; species with higher specific metabolic rates also have a higher age-specific cancer incidence. The faster the rate of aging, the faster accumulation of carcinogenic events, the higher the rate of free-radical production per cell. It is all connected.

One researcher, Richard Cutler, developed an index which associated energy metabolism with aging rates, called the life span energy potential (LEP). The LEP value for a species is defined as the product of its average lifelong specific metabolic rate (SMR), and its maximum life span potential (MLSP). Humans have the highest life span potential, followed by other primates, and then most other mammals. This demonstrates convincingly that aging rate is related to metabolic rate, or the rate of O_2 usage per unit weight of tissue, and this in turn is positively correlated with the rate of ROS production; good evidence to suggest the involvement of ROS as a principal cause of aging!

As important as they are, free radicals are not the sole cause of aging. Many other processes also contribute to the general winding-down of this intricately interconnected system. Aging, by definition, involves a gradual decrease in function. Part of this decrease in function is because the cells in some key tissues are exhausted. They run out of reproductive vigor. Certain tissues, like the ovaries, thymus and pineal glands show a dramatic and catastrophic decline with aging. This involution in the thymus gland is powerfully contributed to by stress hormones, and has in turn, a significant and detrimental effect on the immune system. In young adulthood the ruinous effect that stress hormones have on the thymus gland is counteracted by the endogenous hormone melatonin (MT), but when the pineal gland fails to produce this hormone, there is then nothing to save the thymus gland. In addition, the replacement of essential FAs with saturated fats in the modern diet, as well as overindulgence in t-FAs, has had the effect of hardening our cell membranes, which in turn has leads to cellular senescence, and the consequent failure of cell membranes.

Most of these changes represent symptoms of an organism reaching its limits. Cells were never designed to go on forever, there are limits to cellular reproduction. It may be that these limits do not apply to all tissues, but if they do apply to a few key ones and that is enough to bring the whole cat's-cradle tumbling down. This idea of limits for cellular reproduction was first proposed by August Weissman, more than a century ago.

We have seen that free radicals have a vital role in age-related degeneration. The question now to ask is why? The clear answer that shouts itself at us is that our ancestors did not evolve in an O_2 atmosphere. They were anaerobes. With the exception of our mitochondria our cells are, even today, essential anaerobic. In this sense, working with O_2 is as unnatural to us as it was to our ancestors, 3 billion years ago. They managed to make a compromise to the O_2 in the atmosphere by acquiring mitochondria. If they had not done this, we would never have evolved into the complex creatures that we are today. However, this union was a strained marriage at best. It was a partnership of opposites.

Over the eons, we have adopted certain antioxidant defense systems to help us cope with this poisonous gas, but these are only partial fixes, at best. This deal cut by our ancestors with the mitochondria, 3 billion years ago, contains within it, the seeds of our destruction.

This arrangement hammered out in the muddy pool 3 billion years ago enabled us to walk on the moon, but it also meant that eventually all of the biochemical errors that occur as a result of our dependence on such a reactive chemical as O_2 would eventually catch up with us. It has meant that many cellular functions would over time develop anomalous, erroneous, even aberrant characteristics. It meant that ultimately, the genetic instructions of the cell itself might be altered, and some of the controls that have been built into us over the eons by our evolution, would be overridden.

I can put it no more eloquently than did Karen Reiser: "*Glyco-oxidative damage represents the...Faustian bargain of evolution. The passage from the unconscious immortality of unicellular existence to the complexities of sentient life required the development of an oxidant metabolism, the slow fire that consumes us.*"

CHAPTER 4

MATTERS OF THE HEART

All human history attests
That happiness for man—the hungry sinner—
Since Eve ate apples,
much depends on dinner

Lord Byron

Cardiovascular disease is the leading cause of death in Western countries. In the United States in 1990 nearly 600,000 people died from it. Cardiovascular disease (CVD) is a term for describing all diseases of the heart and blood vessels. It includes Coronary heart disease (CHD), including heart attack and angina pectoris, stroke, and peripheral vascular disease.

The main underlying problem in all of these diseases is a hardening and clogging of the arteries by a process called atherosclerosis.

Atherosclerosis is the leading cause of death and disability in US, UK, and Australia. In all, the number one cause of death is myocardial infarction (MI). The final and sometimes fatal event in CHD, this is a blockage of the coronary artery or its branches.

The risk of CHD increases with age, and is greater for men than for women, for smokers than for non-smokers, for diabetics than for non-diabetics. If you takes a sample of about 5000 men aged 40 from any industrialized country, over one thousand are likely experience a major CHD event before age 65.

The statistics from the USA are representative of other advanced industrial countries. CHD is still the number one killer in the USA, but its incidence is coming down. CHD, and its end point, acute MI, is notably a disease of the our time. At the beginning of the 20th century, acute MI was rare. The incidence of CHD and MI grew slowly between 1920 and 1950, and between 1950 and 1963, it increased markedly. It reached a peak in 1963, when the death rate was 42 percent. The death rate from CHD has declined during each year between 1963 and 1985 except for 1968 and 1980. These two years coincided with epidemics of respiratory disease.

The likely cause of this mortality decline over the last 30 years is the great improvements in prevention and treatment. The death rate from heart disease is still declining, but at a much more modest rate than in the mid 60s. It is possible that with the rise in consumption in packaged and fast food over the past couple of decades that some of the initial gains have been slowed.

In 1990, CHD was responsible for approximately 490,000 deaths in the US, or nearly one in four of the 2.2 million deaths in the US that year. The single leading cause of death is still MI.

Why does CHD increase with age? Does the heart, that most vital of organs fail or become exhausted? Or does it become weakened, due to bad maintenance? Does the fault lie with our hearts, or with us?

The heart like other organs with connective tissue (CT) does weaken with age. Our ability to handle glucose diminishes as we get older, and as they age, most people have their tissues exposed to glucose for longer periods. Higher levels of glucose in the blood most of the time, means that glucose, through its metabolites, AGEs, can react with (cross-link) proteins, and the most common proteins available are those in CT. CT is everywhere, it is the scaffolding upon which our cells rest, and it is present in the heart as well. So with age we can expect to have much more our heart's CT cross-linked than was the case when we were younger.

The fibers of particular importance in the heart are made of the protein elastin. Throughout our lives, there is a constant degradation of these elastin fibers, not only in the heart, but also elsewhere. This is what causes our skin to wrinkle and lose its elasticity. With aging, the elastin fibers in the heart become thinner. This also happens in other tubes that need to stretch, such as the arteries, and the ductus deferens (near the male testicle).

What happens in the heart, is that after it has contracted, the aging heart takes longer to spring back into its normal relaxed position. Because of this, the heartbeat's efficiency is not as good as it was when younger. Additionally, there is another change in the heart with aging, like other muscles, the heart muscle tends to decline in strength with age. This too means that an aging heart is less efficient than a younger one.

However, regrettable as these changes are, in most people they are not responsible for heart attacks. We suffer heart attacks because our heart is denied blood (ischemia). The cause of this condition is not a weak aging heart but a completely different organ. The heart is denied blood because of atherosclerosis, a hardening and blockage of the arteries.

CHD is not so much a disease of the heart, as of the arteries! What is most disappointing about the high death rate from CHD is that of all the diseases, which we are likely to suffer, CHD and stroke are the most likely, and in some ways they are also the most preventable.

There are four independent risk factors associated with CHD and stroke. These are smoking, hypertension or high BP, high blood cholesterol, and physical inactivity. Except for hypertension, all are factors that individuals can change. Other contributors are overweight (obesity), alcohol consumption, and diabetes.

Certain personality traits are also linked to CHD. The incidence of cardiovascular disease as well as deaths from it, tends to be greater among people with less education, less income, and less prestigious jobs or no job.

In order to understand how atherosclerosis arises, we need to study the innermost layer of the artery walls, the endothelium.

The endothelium is the largest organ in the body. In area it is equivalent to six tennis courts, and in mass it is equivalent to five normal hearts (for a 70 kg man). It forms the innermost part of the inner layer of the artery, called the tunica intima. Outside this layer is the tunica media. This is composed mostly of smooth muscle cells (SMCs). This muscle controls the diameter of the arteries, and it this that regulates the blood supply to the tissues, and the BP.

The endothelium, in turn, regulates the tone of this smooth muscle, and therefore has an indirect effect on BP, and the supply of blood to tissues. The endothelium performs its role by producing relaxing and constricting factors, in response to stimuli from the body (physiological), as well as those produced by disease (pathological).

Our blood can form clots. This ability of the blood to clot stops us from bleeding to death when we cut ourselves, and is regulated by clotting factors. The interrelationship of these thrombotic (clot-producing) and anti-thrombotic factors is most of the time, kept in fine balance so that we do not produce clots when we do not need to, but that we have the capacity to make our blood clot, when it is needed.

A healthy endothelial surface maintains blood fluidity. The blood flows well and does not clot unnecessarily. A healthy endothelium has a role in helping the blood to flow well because the endothelial cells secrete a substance called prostacyclin I_2

(PGI_2), which tends to prevent cells in the blood, the platelets, from clumping together to form a clot. PGI_2 is a type of body chemical first derived from the prostate glands of sheep, and therefore called prostaglandins.

The endothelium also produces other chemicals, which cause the smooth muscle in the arteries to constrict (vasoconstriction) and to dilate (vasorelaxation). PGI_2, as well as preventing platelets from aggregating and forming a clot, is a vasorelaxant. This means that it helps the smooth muscle in the artery wall to relax, and that means, that it tends not to narrow, or constrict.

As well, the endothelium produces another substance, endothelium-derived relaxation factor, or EDRF, that causes artery muscle relaxation.

The first event, which triggers CHD is that the endothelium becomes damaged. We are not completely sure what causes this damage. It may be a result of mechanical factors, such as the shear stress of blood being pulsed through the artery, or caused by antigen-antibody complexes. Perhaps it is due to the presence of a blood amino acid, homocysteine, or it may be that a high-fat diet results in the adhesion of phagocytes to the artery lining, which in turn causes damage. Some or all of these factors may be act simultaneously.

Whatever the cause, the surface becomes disturbed. This causes platelets to stick to the surface, and also the release by the endothelium of chemicals, vasoactive amines. These make the endothelial cells leaky, in particular they allow oxidized cholesterol to leak into the space below (outside) the endothelium (the subendothelial space).

It seems that one other factor must also be present for this deadly cascade to get underway. A high concentration of oxidized cholesterol, stimulates macrophages, which consume it in the subendothelial space to become pathological in a way which I will try to explain later. At the same time there is a migration of muscle cells from the tunica media to the tunica intima. Muscle cells thus invade the innermost layer of the artery perhaps in an attempt to heal what the body has perceived as an injury. This all occurs because of an inflammatory reaction in the artery wall.

Inflammation, you will recall, is the response of the immune system to infection or injury. We start this story with damaged endothelial cells. As we have said, these can be damaged by a number of factors.

Cytokines, or chemical messengers, are released at first by the damaged endothelial cells, then by other cells in the area. These stimulate blood flow in the area, and call in growth factors.

Macrophages in the area become very active. They, as well as the endothelial cells, and even some of the SMCs from the artery wall, release a chemical messenger, platelet derived growth factor. Infiltrating macrophages and white cells migrating from the circulation to insinuate themselves in the damaged artery wall secrete a variety of inflammatory- and growth-stimulating local hormones. Platelets and monocytes adhere to the injury site and produce another cytokine, which in turn attracts more lymphocytes, and the disturbed endothelial surface becomes a hive of cells most of which are producing cytokines, chemical messengers, that attract yet more cells to the area.

Very soon at the site of this artery wall disturbance there are a lot of cells all producing chemicals designed to stimulate growth.

This occurs because your immune system sees in your artery wall an open wound that needs to be healed, so all the forces are mobilized to do this. The same events would be called into operation if you cut your finger.

Fibroblasts are attracted to the area to produce CT. Platelets are instructed aggregate to block any holes that can be found, and they also release a chemical which instructs SMCs to migrate from the tunica media to the tunica intima, the inner layer of the artery.

The artery wall has become the site of intense growth-activity. This is atherosclerosis, the result of an inflammatory response. Incidentally, the word atherosclerosis is derived from roots that literally mean hard mush. The hard mush that is being referred to is that atheroma forming in the artery, and that is a fair description of it.

The hard mush is produced by an extensive reaction of the immune system, so that it can be said that when we have a heart attacks, we are being attacked not by our hearts, but by our own immune systems.

What brings about this frantic growth spurt in our artery wall? The traditional view is that high levels of oxidized blood cholesterol are thought to be the principal recruiters of these immune cells. You can make phagocytes adhere to a healthy and intact endothelium simply by feeding the subject with a diet high in oxidized fats.

Injury may also be caused to our endothelium by the amino acid, homocysteine. Some think that viruses are also responsible. Perhaps it is one or more of these factors, alone or together, that triggers this orgy of growth.

If this process continues, an atherosclerotic lesion, an atheroma, will eventually be produced. An atheroma is a type of growth, resembling a mound filled with cells and oxidized cholesterol, in the artery wall. This growth restricts the diameter of the blood vessel, thereby slowing blood flow through the artery. Sometimes the atheroma is so large, that it almost completely blocks the artery.

Since the endothelium is damaged, clotting factors are produced, and clots form. Eventually, the fibrous cap of one of these atheroma breaks, spilling necrotic (dead cells) debris, and thrombotic (clot-producing) substances into the blood stream, along with a large amount of cholesterol. This debris can form a blockage, or it can itself raise a blood clot, which will eventually occlude a branch of the coronary artery of the heart. When a blood clot or debris settles in a branch or branches of the coronary artery already narrowed by the atheroma, the heart muscle experiences ischemia, lack of blood supply, and because the blood supply brings O_2 to (the mitochondria of) the heart, such a heart will then experience anoxia, shortage of O_2.

Ischemia, and the anoxia that results from it, causes a pain, angina pectoris. Sometimes such an ischemic episode results in the death of heart tissue. This is called a heart attack. The tissues of the heart and brain are post-mitotic; they cannot readily be replaced (in an adult) once they die. The death of heart tissue weakens the heart. A strong heart, developed through exercise, and one with plenty of collateral circulation, is in a much better position to survive ischemia.

If the heart has been severely damaged, its pumping ability is immediately depressed, and this results in reduced cardiac output, and damming of blood in the veins. After acute heart attacks, and even sometimes after prolonged periods of slow, progressive cardiac deterioration, the heart becomes incapable of pumping even the minimum amount of blood required to keep the body alive. Consequently, all of the tissues begin to suffer, and even to deteriorate, often leading to death within a few hours, or a few days.

Many people who die of coronary occlusions or myocardial infarctons die because of ventricular fibrillation. This is a generalized but uncoordinated contraction of the ventricle. The tendency to develop fibrillation is especially great, following a large infarction, but fibrillation can follow a small occlusion as well. Indeed some patients with coronary insufficiency die acutely from fibrillation without any noticeable infarction at all.

Atherosclerosis as an inflammatory process is confirmed by the presence of many inflammatory cells, such as lymphocytes, in and around diseased arteries, and also by post-mortem, and in vivo examinations of atherosclerotic plaques. Eighty percent of atherosclerotic sites show a high degree of penetration of lymphocytes, even to the outermost layer of the artery. Those other heralds of the inflammatory process, the mast cells, have also been found in atherosclerotic lesions, as well as in arteries with fatty streaks, the mild beginnings of atherosclerois.

It may be that mast cells promote the formation of early lesions, and they may also participate in atheroma rupture. Mast cells, special immune cells, promote the ingestion of oxidized cholesterol by macrophages. Mast cells in the arteries, both diseased and normal ones, can degrade the apo-HDL, the protein in high-density lipoprotein (HDL).

HDL is the protective form of cholesterol. If the mast cells remove it, we are left only with the disease-causing form of circulating cholesterol, called low-density lipoprotein (LDL).

Another inflammatory processes is the production of antibodies to heat-shock proteins. Heat-shock proteins are the intercellular chaperones, used to stabilize the conformation of other proteins. Many autoimmune and inflammatory conditions are associated with the production of heat-shock proteins. Several heat-shock proteins are found in atherosclerotic lesions.

Atherosclerosis, as an inflammatory process, has other implications. Might it be possible, for example, that viruses and other infectious agents, which we know cause inflammation can also lead to the development of CHD?

In 1983 a research group examined plaques (atheroma) removed in blood vessel surgery, and in 25 percent of their samples they found antigens to the cytomegalovirus (CMV). CMV is a member of the herpes family of viruses, and is very common. A prominent researcher in the area called Malnick has suggested that the CMV might be causing SMCs to proliferate (or to migrate from the tunica media to the tunica intima of arteries). He suggested that if it could be demonstrated that a virus is the cause of these transformations of SMCs, then a vaccine against the virus might prevent atherosclerosis.

Other microorganisms have been implicated in the development of atherosclerosis including the bacteria *Chlamydia pneumoniae*, and perhaps surprisingly, the organisms responsible for periodontal disease, *Propionibacterium Gingivalis*.

Oral hygiene is no trivial matter. More than 300 species of bacteria live in the human mouth. If you sleep with your mouth open, when you wake you have something like several hundred billion bacteria in your mouth. Some can cause serious disease, such as nephritis (inflammation of the kidney) or endocarditis (inflammation of the lining of the heart), and they may also be of prime importance in the inflammatory condition of the artery walls, we call atherosclerosis.

Let's look at what factors initiate this mortal sequence of events. According to the most accepted theory, it all starts with cholesterol, but not just cholesterol on its own. In order to be dangerous, the cholesterol needs to become oxidized, and that is where the prevention comes in. If we can stop that oxidation, we are well on the way to stopping the whole morbid cascade.

Cholesterol is not a bad chemical. It is vital for growth and development of cells in higher organisms. Every cell in our bodies makes it. Evolution does not plan such widespread production of a chemical that is of no use or is only bad.

Chemically, it belongs to a group called sterols, the group which also embraces many of our hormones, such as testosterone, cortisol and estrogen. Indeed, cholesterol is a precursor of those hormones. It is made chiefly by the liver but also by the adrenal glands, and gonads (ovaries and testes).

Cholesterol can be absorbed directly from the diet. It is in the tissues and products of animals, but not present in plants. Egg yolk, fatty meats, liver, and cheese are particularly rich sources.

When you eat cholesterol, the synthesis of further cholesterol by the liver is inhibited. This is because the enzyme, which is responsible for further synthesis, HMG CoA reductase, is inhibited (switched off) by the dietary cholesterol. Therefore having a *little* cholesterol in your diet is not such a bad thing, as it inhibits your own cholesterol production.

The liver is the prime source for most of the body's cholesterol. The liver needs to make heaps of cholesterol for use in the production of bile salts, but some of it is also exported to the tissues. When the liver exports cholesterol, it packs it into lipoprotein particles. These have cholesterol and other lipids on the inside, and an outer coating of lipoprotein.

There are three types of lipoprotein particles, which are classified according to how tightly they are packaged. Cholesterol in the blood normally travels in particular particles that we have already mentioned, LDL and HDL. After being made by the liver and dispatched to the blood, it is packaged in an LDL particle. This is the way that cholesterol travels to the cells.

Upon reaching the target cell, the whole LDL particle is bound to its membrane by means of LDL receptors on the surface, then it is internalized by the cell (surrounded and consumed) by a process called exocytosis; the whole complex, LDL and receptor, is swallowed by the target cell.

The membrane LDL receptor plus the LDL bound to it together migrate to special organelles, lysosomes, where degradation occurs, by means of degradative enzymes. The protein component of LDL is hydrolyzed, to amino acids, and the cholesterol esters are also broken up and used by the cell. The cell then returns the LDL receptor to the membrane for reuse. The round trip lasts 10 minutes. An LDL receptor has a life of one day, and in that time it may bring many LDL particles into the cell.

The LDL receptor is subject to feedback regulation. When cholesterol is abundant inside the cell, new LDL receptors are not synthesized, and the uptake of additional cholesterol from plasma LDL is blocked. Once inside the tissues, cholesterol is used for its variety of functions: to make ear wax, or the outer layer of the skin, or testosterone, or cortisol, or myelin sheaths, and cell membranes.

Excess cholesterol is packaged in the smallest of the lipoprotein particles HDL, and sent back to the liver. Adult humans are peculiar in that they carry 60 to 70 percent of the total cholesterol in their plasma in LDL particles. In newborn human infants, and most adult animals other than man, HDL is the major cholesterol carrier in the plasma.

It is very important to understand this negative feedback regulation, because it is essential in understanding heart disease. If the cholesterol in the blood going to the cells stayed as a typical physiological LDL particle, the negative feedback of the cell would ensure that the cell took only what it needed, and there would be no drama. However, that is not what usually happens. The vital pathological event seems to be that the LDL particle gets oxidized, and that changes everything. Let's look at this.

The LDL particle is a huge spherical molecule. Around the outside of the particle is a tunic of protein. Our cells often recognize particles that are in our bloodstream by the nature of the protein on the surface. If you will, proteins are often used to give a particle an identity. The protein around this particle, called Apolipoprotein B or Apo B, tells the cells that it is an LDL particle and this engages the negative feedback regulation.

So, as long as the cell recognizes the particle as LDL, it will not take too much of it. This is achieved because a cell with the LDL receptor can only absorb LDL, and the LDL receptor is subject to negative feed-back regulation. Where the problem arises that leads to heart disease is when the LDL particle becomes oxidized. This changes the nature of the protein identifier, and the particle is no longer recognized by the regulated LDL receptor anymore, but instead by a different receptor called the scavenger receptor.

This receptor does not have the same feedback control that the LDL receptor has, so when oxidized LDL (oLDL) is encountered by a macrophage, and attaches to its scavenger receptor, the macrophage consumes it, and continues to consume it, until something very strange happens to it. It gets more and more bloated; the oLDL hardens inside it like concrete, and finally it becomes a streak of hard oxidized fat, a fatty streak. This is the first event in hardening of the arteries, arte-riosclerosis.

The LDL particle has 2,200 molecules of cholesterol, also has 2,600 molecules of PUFAs, including LA, Ar. A, and docosahexanoic acids (DHA). These PUFAs are highly susceptible to peroxidation, and so are usually protected by several antioxidants, such as vitamin E and ubiquinol. Each LDL particle carries seven molecules of vitamin E, but also has other antioxidants in much smaller quantities, including alpha-tocopherol (Vitamin E), alpha-carotene, beta-carotene, lycopene, cryp-toxanthine, cantazanthin, lutein, zeaxanthin, phytofluene, retinoids, and coenzyme Q_{10} .

If the levels of these natural antioxidants are low the particle will become oxidized. This oxidation is a lipid peroxidation chain reaction brought about by free radicals but, which requires trace metals supplied by the Fenton reaction. It starts when a free radical removes a hydrogen atom from one of the PUFAs. Free radicals like hydrogen peroxide, the hydroxyl and superoxide radicals, and hypochlorous ions can initiate the reaction, and phagocytes in a respiratory burst can produce these.

A respiratory burst is a deliberate release of free radicals by a phago-cyte to kill an intruder, such as a bacterium. This happens often in our bodies, whenever we have an inflammatory response.

The PUFA oxidation within the LDL particle produces first a PUFA-radical, then a lipid peroxyl radical. This radical takes hydrogen from the next nearest PUFA, creating a new radical, and in this way a chain reaction is established in which hydroperoxides of cholesterol ester are produced.

If enough vitamin E is present, it reacts with the peroxyl radicals, forming tocopheroxyl, which gets converted into something harmless. This is the way that vitamin E can break the chain reaction, and so is called a chain-breaking antioxidant.

If there are not enough antioxidants present, those that are available, compete with lipid molecules for the peroxyl radicals. The lipid hydroperoxides are the initial lipid peroxidation products, these break down to a number of other products, such as aldehydes, epoxides, alcohols, and hydrocarbon gases. These oxidant products, when formed penetrate into the wall of the artery, just below the artery lining, the subendothelial space.

These breakdown products of lipid peroxidation after entering deep within the artery wall are recognized by the scavenger receptors on the tissue macrophages that are stationed there. Once recognized as toxic by the macrophages, they must consume it. The macrophage's scavenger receptor lacks the built in regulation of the LDL-receptor, and they ingest the o-LDL with its toxic breakdown products gluttonously. Some of these breakdown products, such as the lipid aldehydes in o-LDL, are highly cytotoxic.

The macrophage continues to ingest this cytotoxic material until it changes into a lipid-laden cell, called a foam cell. This foam cell, a bloated Goodyear™ blimp of toxic chemicals is not viable. The toxic chemicals within the foam cell eventually harden causing the foam cell to become merely a petrified streak in the artery wall, a fatty streak.

A fatty streak is like a vein of cellular cement. As the fatty streaks continue to accumulate, an atherosclerotic plaque begins to develop. All this migration of macrophages and o-LDL particles into the artery wall causes a lesion or wound in the artery wall. This is made worse by the toxicity of the substances in the o-LDL. These toxic substances continuously release chemicals that irritate the wall of the artery. The open wound within the artery wall becomes more and more irritated, and inflamed, and more and more white cells are called in to help.

This is how o-LDL provokes an inflammatory response-the body's normal reaction to injury. Cytokines are released by the injured endothelium, which acts like an alarm, calling to the area, first macrophages, then later T-cells. Monocytes, already in the area, and those that have been recently summoned there, produce growth factors that stimulate the proliferation of the smooth muscle, and CT in the area of the lesion. SMCs in the artery wall proliferate (multiply) and migrate towards the injury to heal the wound. So what begins as an attempt by the body to heal itself produces a large growth in the artery wall called an atheroma.

This healing process goes wrong because of the toxicity of oxidized lipids in the o-LDL. Antioxidants prevent this fatal oxidant transformation of the LDL.

This is why we should increase our intake of antioxidants, principally vitamin E, but also the ones that regenerate this vitamin, beta-carotene, coenzyme Q_{10} and vitamin C.

Or, to put it in the terms of food, carotenoids (such as beta-carotene) which are found in red-orange vegetables; vitamin C in fresh citrus fruits, potatoes and green vegetables; and vitamin E from cereal seed oils, wheat-germ, margarines and green leafy vegetables. Also needed are bioflavonoids, which also recycle these antioxidants. These are in berries such as mulberry and bilberry, as well as citrus fruit, red capsicums, and buckwheat. These antioxidants act individually and recycle each other. They should therefore be taken together, not individually. Ascorbic acid for example can react with, and scavenge many types of free radicals, including the hydroxyl radical, the superoxide ion and the $1O_2$. In addition, it can regenerate the reduced form of alpha-tocopherol.

Ring structures similar to those found in vitamin E and the phenolics allow these compounds to actively scavenge, and stabilize free radicals. In addition, the presence of carboxylic acid groups in many phenolic compounds can inhibit lipid oxidation by metal chelation-a reversal of the Fenton reaction.

Phenolics are in many foods. These include: vanillin from vanilla beans, and cloves; sesamol from sesame seeds; caffeic acid from oats, soybeans, blueberries, prunes, and grapes; ferulic acid from oats, soybeans, blueberries, prunes and grapes; quercetin from tea, coffee, cereal grains, and onions; epicatechin from tea leaves; epigallocatechin from tea leaves; ellagic acid from grapes, strawberries, and raspberries, and curcumin from turmeric, and mustard.

In addition, there are carnosine and anserine, found in meat, and pyrroloquinoline quinone, widely distributed in microorganisms, plants, and animals.

Consumption of these phenolics has been associated with a reduction in atherosclerosis, and apparent prevention of cancer.

History has many references to the health effects of phenolics. George Washington, for example, would eat boiled onions whenever he felt a cold coming on. What was producing the effect for George was the phenolic quercetin, a natural constituent of onions, as well as asparagus, grapes, apples, citrus rind, and tea.

It helped his cold because it has immune-enhancing effects. It would also have helped to prevent atherosclerosis, and cancer. Much research is being done of quercetin, particularly in Holland. The Dutch eat a lot of onions and apples, natural sources of quercetin, and this is probably why Holland has such a low level of CHD. Smart people! The Dutch.

To understand the important role of antioxidants in forestalling atherosclerosis, it is necessary to look at what has become known at "The French Paradox."

In most countries, such as the UK and the USA for example, high dietary intakes of saturated fat and cholesterol are strongly correlated with mortality from CHD. However in certain regions of France this relationship is less apparent. Mortality rates from CHD in France are closer to those of Japan and China, than those of the USA, or the UK. This finding is paradoxical, given that saturated fat intake in France represents 14 to 15 percent of energy, and serum cholesterol levels are similar to those in the USA and the UK.

This can't be explained by differences in other risk factors for CHD, such as BP, body mass index (BMI), and cigarette smoking. It may, however, be related in part to the regular consumption of red wine, which has various phenolic compounds that impart an astringent taste to it, as well as to tea, coffee, and cocoa. Phenolic compounds include flavonoids, non-flavonoid phenolics, flavanols, and soluble tannins.

It has been proposed that the cardio-protective property of red wine is due to these polyphenols. Why red wine and not white? Polyphenols are in the skin of the grape. Red wine, when being made, is in contact with the grape skins longer than white wine, and so absorbs more of the polyphenols.

It may be that the French are doing more than one thing right! The French diet is also high in vegetable oils, and this means that they also have a higher intake of vitamin E, than do, say, the British. So probably it is both of these dietary protectors that are helping the French.

Vegetable oil and red wine consumption is common throughout most of the southern Europe, a legacy of the ancient Greeks and Romans. Italy, Greece, France, and Portugal, all have comparatively low levels of CHD; much lower than their cousins who have migrated to the New World, the US, and Australia, and lower than in Britain. So perhaps the French Paradox should be called the Mediterranean Paradox.

In fact, we do know a bit more about the protective diets of the Mediterranean people than we did in 1992, when Renaud and De Lorgeril, published their important paper on the French Paradox.

A diet high in olive is associated with low levels of cholesterol, blood glucose, and BP. Cretans, who drink olive oil from a glass, like wine, have very low levels of CHD, because olive oil, with its monounsaturated FAs, raises the levels of the 'good' cholesterol or HDL, while causing no significant increase in the 'bad' cholesterol or LDL. But if you are trying to lose weight, and you do not work as hard as the agrarian workers of Crete, this might not be such a good idea, since all fats contain the same high levels of energy. As well, a diet high in olive oil has also been found to be protective against breast cancer in Italy and in Greece.

So it seems that if you want to live long and prosper, you should adopt a diet like that popular in Southern Europe, plenty of olives and/or olive oil, tomatoes, beans, garlic, onions, carrots, and, of course, red wine. I am all for that!

The Japanese have a diet which is very low in vitamin E, and they do not have as much grape wine as Southern Europeans, but they have one of the lowest levels of CHD in the developed world. This is in spite of having many other CHD risk factors, such as a very high rate of smoking.

A possible explanation for this is that the Japanese eat a lot of fish. Increased fish consumption is protective against CHD and stroke, even in heavy smokers.

There is an enormous amount of literature attesting to the cardio-protective effect of fish consumption. There are at least three con-stituents in fish that are likely to have a good effect. Fish have a high level of Se used in an important antioxidant enzyme system. They also have a predominance of N-3 FAs that prevent platelets from sticking together, and thereby forming clots. As well, people on high-fish diets tend to have less homocysteine. Methionine, the precursor of homo-cysteine, is more common in red meat than in fish.

Another of our antioxidant defenses is the seleno-protein GPX. The protective effect of the antioxidant Se is demonstrated by the Sami peo-ple, who are Laps living in northern Finland. Unlike other Fins, they have a relatively low incidence of CHD. Living in the cold northerly extremes of Sweden and Finland, they have a diet mostly of fish and reindeer. Luckily for the Sami, each of these foods is high in an impor-tant antioxidant. The reindeer is high in vitamin E and fish is high in Se. The Samis, like other Fins, are heavy smokers, and also have high levels of cholesterol, but like the French and Japanese their diet is high in antioxidants, which affords them sufficient protection notwithstand-ing other risk factors.

What seems to be enabling the Sami to beat the odds, is a plentiful supply of Se. When it is plentiful, the GPX system is works well. Se is one of the most important antioxidants. When someone has a serious infection, say HIV, their antioxidants fall, because they are being used quenching the free radicals produced by the phagocytes. Se levels fall significantly in HIV-infected people.

When they are further infected, as they usually are because HIV attacks the immune system, the levels of Se fall even more. Se also seems to be very good at preventing the damage to DNA caused by toxic agents, which often precedes cancer.

Too much Se though is poisonous. People who have excessive Se in their drinking water do suffer its toxic effects, and sometimes also devel-op a serious neurological disorder called amyotrophic lateral sclerosis (ALS). Having issued that warning let me add that many people do take

Se under the guidance of a qualified health professional, and do very well.

When evidence of the relationship between dietary antioxidant intake and CHD mortality was evaluated, vitamin E intake appeared to be inversely related to the risk of death from CHD. This relationship was especially striking in the subgroup of 21,809 women who had not previously taken vitamin supplements. Impressive though these studies were, they weren't clinical trials. Such trials are under way.

Such strongly positive findings from these three studies, each with a large group of subjects, are pretty convincing. One of these studies also established an association between CHD, and the intake of vitamin C and beta-carotene, as well as vitamin E.

This research adds to the growing evidence that strongly suggests that antioxidants, especially fat-soluble antioxidants such as vitamin E, may protect against atherosclerosis by reducing the generation of o-LDL cholesterol. They also confirm similar findings from other studies, not so large, such as the Zutphen Elderly Study which found high intakes of flavonoids associated with lower CHD mortality in a sample of 805 elderly men, and the Euramic study, in which beta-carotene was found to be protective against myocardial infarction in a sample of 1410 subjects in nine countries.

These are only some of the many studies involving the amelioration of CHD by vitamin E and other antioxidants, many others are available.

Another cholesterol particle already mentioned is HDL, which some call 'good cholesterol'. People who have high levels of it are less likely to suffer from CHD, and, when they do, it is often less severe. Women have higher levels of HDL than men, and a lower risk of CHD. HDL is a specially sized package of cholesterol (esters) by which cholesterol is sent back to the liver from the tissues-called the reverse cholesterol transport. This process daily may transfer one gram of cholesterol daily.

HDL can strip LDL-cholesterol (bad cholesterol) from your arteries. How? It seems that it can enter vessel walls, although how it does this is not known. Lipoproteins are composed of a lipid-core surrounded by a protein coat, as we saw with LDL. The protein in HDL is called apo-A1, or apo-lipoprotein A1. This protein has a high affinity for cholesterol. It can't get enough of it, and will grab it from anywhere. When

HDL gets into the tissues therefore, it binds with the cholesterol (cholesterol ester). It can even bind with cholesterol in the intima of the arteries, where it takes part in a limited type of reversal of atherosclerosis.

HDL can be oxidized in the same way that LDL is oxidized and when it is it is no longer able to perform reverse cholesterol transport. Yet another reason to take sufficient antioxidants. How can I increase my levels of HDL? A good start is to have the right genes. About 50 percent of the chance of having either high HDL or high LDL is down to our genes. Cholesterol (lipoprotein) disorders are due to an abnormality in the synthesis, breakdown, or processing of cholesterol (lipoprotein) particles (LDL and HDL). More than half of the people with lipoprotein disorders, and atherosclerosis before the age of 60, have a familial lipoprotein disorder.

Is there anything that I can do to increase my HDL other than being born in the right family? HDL levels are moderately increased by weight loss. Elevated triglycerides usually appear with low HDL, so there might be a link between these two, so if you lower your triglycerides, then your HDL should rise. People with familial lipoprotein disorders have a fourfold chance of having both an elevated triglyeride level, and a low HDL level. Triglycerides are an independent risk factor for CHD, but the relationship between high triglyceride levels and CHD is not clear. Very high levels of CHO in the diet increase triglyceride levels, and high levels of triglycerides go hand in hand with low levels of HDL. On the other hand, high levels of monounsaturated FAs, the ones found in olive and canola oils, tend to increase the levels of HDL, while having little or no effect on the LDL. Smoking reduces levels of HDL. Increased physical activity is thought to raise HDL and lower triglycerides. The vitamin niacin or nicotinic acid lowers LDL and triglycerides, and raises HDL, when administered in doses 100-fold over those required to treat deficiencies in this vitamin (pellagra). Such a dose, building up gradually to 4 grams per day may cause flushing in the face, and other parts of the body, because it opens the small blood vessels. This treatment is not recommended for people with hypertension (high BP).

Finally, HDL is affected by alcohol intake. Apo A1 is synthesized mainly in the liver, and its synthesis is stimulated by alcohol intake, irrespective of the source of the alcohol.

Some early oral versions of the contraceptive pill (OC) have been associated with cardiovascular disease. As early as 1961, a case of pulmonary emboli attributed to the pill was reported. In 1962, the pill was associated with stroke.

In subsequent years, the administration of hormonal contraceptives was reported to be a risk factor for several vascular problems. This trend associating increased mortality from cardiovascular disease with the use of OC continued through out the 1970s, and was supported by several important studies. The most extensive of these was that of the Royal College of General Practitioners, that of the Oxford Family Planning Association, and the Kaiser Permanente Walnut Creek Prospective Contraceptive Study. The three main vascular problems linked with the use of combined hormonal contraceptives were venous thrombo-embolism, thrombotic stroke, and myocardial infarction, or coronary thrombosis. However, Shearman criticized this data in 1981. He made the point that OC predisposed only to certain forms of cardiovascular disease and only in women aged 35 years or more, while it was mostly young women that use the pill.

There have been many changes in OC formulation over the years, and in its recommended use. In one study, in which 65,000 healthy women were examined, it was shown that the taking of the OC correlated with the incidence of venous thrombo-embolism, through the periods from 1977 to 1979, and 1980 through 1982. In the latter period, the risk to women who took the pill was nearly threefold. For both periods, there had been no association between OC use and stroke or myocardial infarction.

Two subsequent studies have been even more reassuring concerning the occurrence of fatal conditions in healthy OC users. In 50,000 woman-years of observation among women aged 15 to 44 who used the pill between the years 1977 to 1982, there was no significant evidence of OC use on mortality. In general, it seems that this decrease in the association between OC and cardiovascular disorders in the USA is due to:

1) the decrease in the dosage of estrogen in OC;
2) the selection of the healthiest women to receive OC;
3) the use of OC before the age of 35 years.

Recent data suggest that there was an increase in the incidence of cardiovascular disease and mortality only in OC users older than 35, and among those who smoked. The use of the pill containing less than 50 micrograms estrogen does not appear to be associated with an increased risk of cardiovascular disease in healthy, non-smoking women, even those 35 to 45 years. It is becoming clear that the combined use of tobacco and OC does contribute substantially to the excess cases of myocardial infarction among US women aged 35 to 44. The risk of these two behaviors combined increases the risk synergistically.

Cholesterol and o-LDL are important in the development of CHD, but there is no one explanation of how this disease develops. o-LDL must only be one cause of atherosclerosis, because up to two-thirds of heart attack survivors do not have high levels of cholesterol in their blood.

Fats are not the only dietary factor of importance in the prevention of CHD, also of importance are proteins, as are the amino acids (AAs), of which the proteins are composed. For example, the AA arginine is very important for the endothelial synthesis of nitric oxide, which may relax our arteries and thereby help to maintain a healthy BP. Glutathione, an important antioxidant, is made up of three amino acids, cysteine, glycine, and glutamic acid.

One of the 20 essential amino acids is methionine. Animal proteins are rich in methionine. Methionine serves an important function in the liver. It, and its metabolite s-adenosyl-methionine, is used as a source of methyl groups for the hepatic transamination vital to protein storage and NH3 management. It is also important to have sufficient methyl donors such as methionine available, for the maintenance of healthy DNA.

When methionine gives up a methyl group, it is converted to homocysteine. This is a reversible reaction, and, in the liver after demethylation, the homocysteine is converted back to methionine by a reaction that requires vitamin B_{12}, folic acid, and vitamin B_2, and vitamin B_6, as cofactors. About 77 percent of the homocysteine produced in the liver is safely re-methylated back to methionine in this way.

Endothelial cells, which line our arteries, lack the enzyme necessary to metabolize methionine safely. A high concentration of methionine in the endothelial cells therefore, results in a high concentration of homocysteine. This problem is more frequent among the Caucasian race than among others. Black people are more efficient at metabolizing methionine, and this may explain why they have lower levels of CHD.

High levels of homocysteine have been shown to cause atherosclerosis in animals, and as between 20 to 40 percent of humans with CHD also have elevated levels of homocysteine suggests that it is very likely that homocysteine is a contributor to atherosclerosis in humans as well. Methionine, the precursor of homocysteine, damages the endothelium of animals, and methionine-loading in humans causes loss of endothelial cells. Is it methionine, or homocysteine, that causes damage to arteries? We do not know!

Methionine does not seem to be a problem in the liver, where it can be safely re-methylated from homocysteine. It is likely that methionine is merely the precursor for the really toxic chemical, homocysteine. If you take some cells from the aorta and expose them to homocysteine you kill them instantly. Furthermore, it does not happen only in the laboratory. We know that homocysteine is poisonous to our arteries. After the poisoning and loss of the endothelial cells by homocysteine exposure, all of the inflammatory atherosclerotic events described for o-LDL take place.

Homocysteine also interferes with clotting. Blood clotting is a complicated process, with a vast interplay of pro- and anti- clotting factors. To have too many of the clotting factors is not a good thing, since it will result in a clot which can block (occlude) an artery in the heart, brain, or somewhere else. But equally, with too few clotting factors, we could bleed to death, as can hemophiliacs, who have a lifelong clotting disorder inherited from their mothers.

Endothelium has qualities that prevent unnecessary clotting. The first of these is its smooth surface. This is what gets disturbed o-LDL and homocysteine. The second is a layer of glycoproteins called glycocalyx, which lines the endothelium. This layer tends to inhibit clotting and can become disturbed by the cells and toxins involved in atherosclerosis. The third is a chemical produced by the endothelium itself: an endothelial anti-clotting factor called thrombomodulin.

This protein binds to the thrombin, the pro-clotting enzyme in the blood, inactivating it. Homocysteine inhibits the production of thrombomodulin by the endothelium allowing the clotting process goes into top gear.

How does homocysteine cause damage to the endothelium? It acts like a free radical, and probably also generates H_2O_2. The cytotoxic mechanism of homocysteine is mediated by the -SHs, which the molecule carries, and is accelerated by transition metals, as are most oxidant reactions.

Sulfur is in the same group of the Periodic Table as oxygen, so -SH could be expected to have similar properties to -OH, and we know that -OH can become the hydroxyl radical, so perhaps something similar is happening involving -SH.

We know that homocysteine toxicity can be neutralized by the presence of CAT-an enzyme that renders H_2O_2 harmless. So, perhaps the toxicity of homocysteine is mostly by its generation of H_2O_2.

Oxidant stress is the main cause of an imbalance between methionine and homocysteine, and the process seems to be catalyzed by those dangerous transition metals, in this case copper.

How can the accumulation of homocysteine in our arteries be prevented? The reaction that transforms methionine into homocysteine is accelerated in an oxidant environment, which allows the release of transition metals from their normal binding to proteins, so we need to take antioxidants to produce a reducing environment-not one of oxidation.

As well, folic acid (folate) will drive the reaction towards the production of methionine, and away from producing toxic homocysteine. So we need to take folate, and because folate is aided by vitamin B_{12}, it is a good idea to combine your folate therapy with it. All women and girls of childbearing age should take 0.5 mg of folate a day to avoid the possibility of neural-tube defect. Older people should take folate as well, to avoid homocysteine-induced atherosclerosis.

For the best results, you should take vitamin B_{12} with the folate, but B_{12} taken orally requires a cofactor, called intrinsic factor, to be absorbed. The stomach produces intrinsic factor in limited amounts.So the maximum amount of B_{12} that can be absorbed after oral administration is limited by the available intrinsic factor.

There is a way around this, and that is to take your B_{12} sublingually. B_{12} can be taken under the tongue and be absorbed directly into the blood from the mucous membrane. When absorbed this way, it does not require intrinsic factor.

The other cofactor required to drive your homocysteine back to methionine is vitamin B_6. Supplementation with modest amounts of these vitamins results in a significant reduction in homocysteine levels.

Overweight individuals are twice as likely to develop CHD than people of normal weight. An early researcher into weight and health, Quetelet, realized that among people of normal build but different heights, weight was proportional to height squared. This observation has been broadened into a clinical tool for use with adults, already mentioned, BMI.

$$BMI= weight (kg)/height (m)2$$

As BMI increases, so too do the chances of having high levels of blood lipids, high BP, and CHD. When BMI exceeds 25 (see Table 1), the risk of death from all causes increases. The principal cause of this is insulin resistance. Overweight is one risk factor for CHD. Another, also associated with body weight, is the fat distribution.

Central obesity (a pot belly, central or intra-abdominal obesity) is a significant risk factor for CHD in men and post-menopausal women. This is independent of body weight. Central obesity is a powerful risk factor because it is associated with visceral obesity, or fat around the organs. Visceral fat breaks down into blood lipids more readily than fat deposits in other parts of the body.

A person with central obesity is apple-shaped, or android. The shape more characteristic of pre-menopausal women is a pear-shape. In pre-menopausal women, fat tends to be deposited on the hips, buttocks, and thighs, rather than on the belly. This shape is referred to as gynoid. It is not that simple though. There is crossover between the sexes, not all men are android, some are gynoid, and not all women are gynoid, some are android.

Table 1: Grades of obesity

BMI	Grade of obesity
0-20	Underweight
20-24.9	Normal weight
24.9-29.9	Overweight
30-39.9	Moderately obese
Over 40	Severely obese

Because android obesity is associated with a greater CHD risk than does gynoid obesity, another index of measurement has been created, called the wasit:hip ratio (WHR). This is obtained by dividing the circumference of the waist by the circumference of the hip. A WHR equal to or less than 0.95 in men, or equal to or less than 0.8 in women is acceptable. Higher ratios indicate health risk.

Not only is increased central or visceral fat a strong risk factor for CHD, it is also for many other disorders, including NIDDM, breast cancer, stroke, and overall mortality, irrespective of weight in general. The other significant risk factors are smoking and high BP (hypertension).

Smoking is particularly good at producing many of the important factors for atherosclerosis. Nicotine causes free-radical formation and lipid peroxidation, and also causes the endothelial cells to become permeable to large molecules such as fibrinogen (the protein that causes clotting).

In humans, you can see abnormalities in the endothelium of umbilical cord vessels from smoking mothers, as compared with non-smoking mothers.

Smoking causes a decrease in HDL. It leads to blood clotting by causing an imbalance between PGI_2 and thromboxane in the artery wall, and by stimulation platelet activation. An atherosclerotic plaque usually must be disrupted before it can cause a complete blockage. This disruption results in thrombus (or clot) formation. There is a lot in cigarette smoke that stimulates clot formation, including the activation of the coagulation and platelet system, and increasing fibrinogen.

Nicotine is a drug, and one of the pharmacological effects of it is that it causes constriction in all arteries, including those that supply the heart. Indeed, the coronary artery has been found to narrow after a single cigarette. It is not only the nicotine that is harmful in cigarette smoke, it is also the carbon monoxide, and another 4000 constituents.

There are many studies linking cigarette smoking with CHD morbidity and mortality. In the 1950s, a study of 187,783 men noted that smokers showed a 52 percent excess in mortality from CHD. A British study in the 1970s, involving 34,000 men, again showed a marked increase in CHD among smokers, as did the Framingham Heart Study.

The 1980s saw major studies involving women for the first time, such as the Nurses' Health Study, which showed that the risk increased by more than five times for the heaviest smokers. Factors relating to CHD, other than CHD morbidity and mortality, were also studied. One group in the 1970s found significantly greater coronary atherosclerosis in smokers compared to non-smokers, as did autopsies from the Honolulu Heart Study.

Giving up smoking lessens the risk of death and disability from CHD. According to Goldman and Cook over half the decline in CHD-related mortality that has occurred since 1968 could be attributed to reductions in cholesterol and cigarette smoking. Indeed, 24 percent of the decline in CHD mortality from 1968 to 1976 has been attributed to the cessation of cigarette smoking alone.

There have been major studies done on this, covering 12 million men and women over four decades. The results are all the same: the cessation of smoking rapidly results in a reduction of thrombogenic effects (blood clot making danger), as well as in the progression of atherosclerosis. These benefits apply both to people who have CHD and those who do not.

Hypertension, which is known to be influenced by genetic factors, is also a risk factor for CHD. The average BP as well as the prevalence of hypertension both tend to rise progressively with increasing age. Estimates from the National Health and Nutrition Examination Survey (NHANES III) tell us that approximately one in four adult residents of the United States has hypertension, with a similar effect seen in other industrialized countries. According to this report, the prevalence of hypertension ranged from 4 percent in young adults, aged 18 to 29, to 65 percent for those 80 years old and older. In youth and middle age men tend to have more hypertension than women.

There are some societies, which have low average BPs, and which do not show age-related changes in it. These tend to be isolated communities, physically active ones, and ones in which the members have a natural diet, low in sodium and potassium. These communities are very interesting, because they tell us that an increase in BP with age is not inevitable, and that the increases in BP that we do see associated with aging are at least to some extent, avoidable. It may be that as we came to live in highly industrialized societies and ate processed foods, containing a relatively high sodium to potassium ratio, we experienced more stress, got fat, and as a consequence experienced this age-related increase in hypertension.

A large number of prospective studies have linked progressively higher levels of systolic and diastolic BP with myocardial infarction, as well as with stroke, congestive heart failure, and renal insufficiency. Because hypertension is a CHD risk, and is associated with aging, older people should have their BPs taken regularly. If they have hypertension (defined as a diastolic measurement over 90 mm of Hg), they should consider medication, in consultation with their doctor.

Other lifestyle changes that may help are weight reduction, increased physical activity, moderation in alcohol consumption, and perhaps a decrease in dietary sodium. In BP treatment the aim should be to maintain a systolic equal to or below 140 mm Hg, and a diastolic equal to or below 90 mm Hg.

One of the factors leading to higher levels of CHD as we age is the fact that as we do so, we become less physically active. Nearly 60 percent of adults in the US are defined as sedentary. Similar figures would apply to other industrialized communities, such as those in Australia, Canada and Western Europe. A sedentary life style is defined as engaging in little, or only irregular, physical activity.

Many epidemiological studies relate physical activity with a decrease in fatal and nonfatal heart disease. Further, exercise is associated with a lower coronary risk, even in old age, and irrespective of other risk factors. So a smoker who exercises is better off than one who does not.

Physical activity was found to decrease the cholesterol-related coronary risk in both elderly men and women, as demonstrated in the NHANES I study.

We are not sure of how regular exercise lowers CHD risk, but we do know a few of the benefits. Exercise increases HDL cholesterol; lowers triglycerides; reduces body fat; reduces fibrinogen; helps to maintain normal glucose tolerance; reduces the tendency for platelets to aggregate (and form a clot); promotes an increased diameter in the coronary arteries; improves the efficiency of the heart's electrical stability and its contraction, and develops additional collateral circulation within the heart itself. It brings about a reduction in the rate of coronary artery atherosclerosis, and reduces body weight, which is in it a risk factor, and it acts as a counterbalance to other less sensible behaviors and habits. Exercise is terrific!

To get all of these benefits though, you need to keep physically fit, and that means work. Both males and females of any adult age can enjoy benefits in relation to CHD from regular exercise. Exercise increases the O_2 supply to the heart muscle and decreases O_2 demand. It makes the heart more efficient.

Physically fit people have a lowered heart rate and BP at rest, and a general reduction in sympathetic tone, which refers to the fact that during and immediately after exercise their heart rate is not as high as it would be in an unfit person doing the same amount of work. If your heart is efficient, as it will be if you are physically fit, then the muscles are getting enough O_2, for comparatively little work. It is therefore harder for them to become ischemic.

Some people think that exercise is dangerous, and they are not entirely wrong. Sudden death from a heart attack does sometimes occur immediately after strenuous exercise, usually, when the person is at rest after stopping acute vigorous activity. Such deaths are usually associated with people who suddenly and vigorously exercise at a time when they are not used to it. For exercise to benefit you, you need to start slowly, building intensity gradually, preferably under the guidance of a qualified person. The aim is to become fit, not dead!

One group of researchers led by Mittelman, interviewed 1,228 patients who had survived heart attacks and examined their behavior before them. They found that, yes, there was a much higher risk of heart attack after heavy exertion, but also that those men who exercised regularly had the lowest risk. Another study at a large hospital in Berlin came to the same conclusion. Exercise can be a trigger for a heart attack, but mostly in those who do not exercise regularly. Physical exercise will protect you, but only if it is regular.

So what is a primary prevention lifestyle strategy for the prevention of CHD? As for diet, we can do little better than follow a diet typical of Southern Europe, rather than one more typical of the US, UK, and Australia, and to paraphrase St. Paul's advice to Timothy, take a little wine, not only for your stomach's sake, but also for the sake of your heart.

It is important to cut down on saturated fats-usually processed and fast foods but also full-cream dairy foods. Things such as pre-made dips also have high levels of fats. The fat content of fast foods is often compounded because preparation involves repeated frying in vats containing (oxidized) oil.

We should increase our intake of seafood, particularly oily or cold-water fish, such as salmon, and mackerel, but also sardines and tuna, to increase our levels of N-3 PUFAs.

We should be sparing in our use of butter and of margarine. Butter is high in SaFAs, as is cheese. Margarine contains unnatural PUFAs and t-FAs, which also should be limited.

We can take liberal amounts of olive and canola oils.

We should increase our intake of fruit and vegetables.

We should take vitamin E at 400 iu a day, and makes sure that our diet is high in vitamin C.

We should have our BP and cholesterol levels taken regularly.

We should lose weight, give up smoking, and, try to control stress in our lives, for instance by meditation, or progressive relaxation exercises.

We should take regular exercise-preferably 20 minutes of good aerobic exercise at least three times a week. It can be jogging, swimming, cycling (with or without lateral movement), brisk walking, or structured aerobic classes. If unused to exercise, undertake a gradual and monitored program.

Also, always allow at least two hours to pass between eating and exercise.

For some people, the lipid levels do not come down even when they follow the program outlined above. They have genes that make that their bodies are less efficient at dealing with lipids, and they require pharmacological intervention under the supervision of a doctor.

Psychological factors can be contributors to CHD. The word "stress" is derived from the word "distress," which in turn is derived from the Old French word estresse, meaning oppression. During the Middle Ages, the term also meant "the pressure exerted by an object."

In 1897, Sir William Osler, a leading professor of Medicine at the end of the 19th century, was the first to link stress with CHD, when he said: *"in the worry and strain of modern life, arterial degeneration is not only very common but develops at a relatively early age. For this I believe that the high pressure at which men live and the habit of working the machine to its maximum are responsible...."*

Two San Franciscan cardiologists, Meyer Friedman and Ray Roseman, invented the idea of the Type A Behavior Pattern (TABP) in 1959. This was a profile of behavior, which they expected might predispose the possessor to CHD. It was further refined in 1974.

Such a person was described as being aggressively involved in the chronic, incessant struggle to achieve more and more in less and less time. Ten years later, the concept was refined still further, offering a more psychodynamic model, and creating a questionnaire that could be used in a clinical setting.

A number of studies have attempted to see if most people suffering from CHD really do have TABP. The first large-scale prospective investigation was the Western Collaborative Group Study. It found that men classified Type A had approximately twice the incidence of CHD as those without that type of behavior (Type B). The Framingham Heart Study, conducted seven years later, came to a similar conclusion. However in later data, such as that from the Framingham Study, the only connection with a Type A personality that was found was with angina pectoris (pain caused by cardiac ischemia) and not with the more serious conditions, such as fatal coronary events. Several other studies, the Multicenter Post-Infarction Research Program; the Aspirin Myocardial Infarction Study, and the Multiple Risk Factor Intervention Trial, all found no relationship between the TABP and CHD in populations at high risk.

One of the groups who earlier had suspected a relationship, the Western Collaborative Group Study, did a follow-up almost ten years later, and found that individuals who had been diagnosed Type A in 1960, and who had developed CHD had only about half the mortality of those diagnosed Type B in the intervening 23 years. So rather than being a risk factor, this group wondered if having a Type A personality might actually be protective.

The personality factor that has in fact had the strongest connection with heart disease is anger. Anger, which derives from the Icelandic word, angr, meaning grief or sorrow, is the state of being at war with oneself, and so with others. Nothing is more damaging to body or mind. It is right to feel angry when someone has done something dreadful to you. You feel angry, take some retributive action, and then it is over. That is perfectly normal and natural. The type of anger, which is destructive, is the smoldering resentment that can last for years, even a lifetime. This is the sort of anger that does harm.

One group of researchers recently tried a number of interventions, designed to make their subjects stressed or angry. Of all the conditions, it was anger that elicited the greatest impairment of heart function, with seven out of the 18 subjects showing a drop in the amount of blood ejected in a contraction of the left ventricle.

Many studies have associated CHD with hostility. In 1987, Williams coined the term hostility complex to describe a type of behavior that correlated strongly to CHD. He described hostility complex as being marked by a cynical, untrusting, and pessimistic attitude to interpersonal relationships, and to life in general. In operation, the hostility complex is measured by the Ho (hostility) scale on the Minnesota Multiphasic Personality Inventory.

Among a group of Western Electric employees, initially healthy, low Ho scores were associated with the lowest incidence of CHD over the subsequent 10-year period. Similar results were found after a 28-year follow-up study on a group of law students. It has to be said also, that a number of other studies failed to find a relationship between Ho scores and CHD morbidity and mortality. Why are there inconsistencies? Questionnaire studies are very hard to keep valid, as individuals are reluctant to admit to what they perceive as personality failings, and/or socially undesirable characteristics, such as hostility.

As well, some people are unaware of the extent of their hostility, and, in certain circumstances, such as job or psychological interviews, people often suppress their hostility, and have low Ho scores.

One other psychosocial factor that has an impact on CHD is social support, or the degree to which an individual is connected to others. This has emerged as a risk factor for morbidity and mortality from many causes, not just CHD. Social support seems to be the strongest psychosocial factor in relation to influence from the mind on CHD.

One group claim that social support is a more important risk factor in relation to CHD than is cigarette smoking. Another finds the most protective factor against CHD is feelings of being loved. That is not hard to understand- the need to be loved is the greatest of human needs.

Having functional and supportive relationships also prolongs the life of people after they have suffered a heart attack, and the author of one of these studies, in an editorial, urges physicians and others to consider social support networks for isolated cardiac patients.

Can my job kill me? It might, if you have the wrong sort of job. One where you have a lot of pressure, and importantly, little say about how it is to be performed. One researcher looked at the results from 37 studies published between 1981 and 1993, and concluded that most of these found a significant correlation between job strain and both CHD and CHD-mortality. Indeed, job stain correlates with all-cause mortality, so, yes; your job might kill you.

We cannot be sure to what extent recent catastrophic events can lead to coronary mortality. There have been many reports of increases in CHD-mortality in the weeks or months following natural or man-made disasters, such as civil war and earthquakes, but there is not universal agreement. The impact of such disasters is hard to judge scientifically, because there is such a huge interplay of events and forces.

Perhaps it is better to say that substantial personal stress and/or bereavement arising from the disaster can be the major contributor to the onset of CHD and CHD-mortality. One group found that widowed men had a significantly higher mortality from CHD in the first six months after their bereavement, than did married men of the same age.

People can die of a broken heart. We see examples all the time. Another group obtained a similar finding, but it suggested that the mortality was higher later, rather than sooner, after the bereavement. However, such relationships are far from clear. Indeed, the evidence for death to follow bereavement is stronger than to death specifically from CHD.

Notwithstanding that however, it is clear from reviewing the literature on the subject, that stress and anxiety arising from many causes, have been statistically linked the risk of CHD, in a large number of studies. Thus it has to be said, that stress seems to be a significant factor in the development and results of CHD, however, the relationship is not as clear as some people might like to think. It must be added that one's attitude to catastrophic events is of primary importance in how destructive life-changing happenings, such as, divorce, unemployment, and even bereavement are going to be to you.

Sudden death is a serious problem within industrialized societies, causing, for example, 400,000 fatalities a year in the US. It usually, but not always happens to people who already have a serious cardiac condition. Usually, the cause of death is a lethal tachyarrhythmia (a fast but irregular series of contraction by the a ventricle). Although rare, there have been reports of life-threatening arrhythmias following severe psychological stress in healthy people. Examples of the types of experiences, which preceded this reaction, were interpersonal conflicts, public humiliation, threat of or actual marital separation, bereavement, and nightmares. You can drop dead after a fright, or a fight.

A relationship between the mind and the heart has been suspected since that extraordinary classical period in Greece. Both Plato and Hippocrates spoke of it. The fact that psychological factors can cause physiological changes was noted early in the 20th century. Since then, a large body of evidence has been accumulated that can be called cardiac psychology.

If I can indulge myself with a personal story, I would like to tell you about my late, and beloved, grandmother. She did not have much in the way of secondary education. I was a high-school student, when she told me that the heart was the source of the emotions, and that emotional turmoil could upset the heart. "Rubbish Grandma," I said, "Your heart is just a pump, and nothing else." She looked a bit confused, but said nothing. I hadn't tried to tell her how to suck eggs, but I had thought that I knew more about physiology than she did, even when I was in high school.

It has taken me many years to realize that there was a good deal of truth in what Grandma said. Follow my Grandma's advice: cultivate positive thoughts, and be careful of the emotions that you let yourself experience; continually monitor them, because emotions are matters of the heart.

CHAPTER 5

CONFRONTING THE CRAB

Under the Greeks, Hippocrates was the first to use the term carcinoma (karkinoma), and he likened cancer to the crab because of its tenacious ability to spread.

Harry Keil

Bulletin of the History of Medicine, 1950; 24: 352-77

As we get older, in one way or another we all confront the crab. All of us will often experience the type of genetic damage which might under some conditions, turn into abnormal cellular behavior. Our genes are fragile, and this was something recognized early by the Universe, which equipped us with fail-safe devices for repairing genetic damage. If we are really unlucky; if we have a particular genetic predisposition against the suppression of this disease; if we come into contact with certain noxious chemicals in high concentration; or if we are subjected to lots of oxidant stress and our antioxidant defenses are run down or overwhelmed; we may acquire this disease, the disease of the crab, cancer.

Cancer is unrestrained cellular growth. The word tumor, which means a growth, comes for the Greek word tymbos meaning a sepulchral mound, and from the Latin word tumere, which means to swell.

Tumor cells, which are also sometimes called neoplastic (from the Greek meaning something newly formed or molded cells, can be divided broadly into two categories, benign and malignant. All tumor cells are cells, which reproduce true to type, and are ones in which the usual controls on reproduction fail to operate.

Benign tumors tend to stay at their place of origin. There are many types and they are usually harmless, but sometimes benign tumors growing in certain vital organs can so disrupt the organ's activity that they become fatal. Benign tumors retain some of the characteristics of the tissue from which they originate, and are classified according to that tissue. Papillomas, keratomas, pigmented moles, and warts, are all skin tumors, with different characteristics depending on the particular type of skin cell from which they arose.

Malignant tumors do not stay localized in their tissue of origin. They invade and destroy surrounding normal tissues by detaching small groups of cells, which then travel (or metastasize) through the blood or lymphatic circulation to other sites distant from the site of origin.

Malignant tumors have two categories, the carcinoma, and the sarcoma. Carcinomas are cancers of epithelial cells, which are cells that line the outer and inner surfaces of the body. Sarcomas arise from the cells of the CT, such as bone, cartilage, tendons, muscles, and the lymphatic system. Although there is five times more CT in the body than epithelial tissue, carcinomas are responsible for about 85 percent of all cancers in adults. The rate of sarcomas remains constant with aging, but carcinomas increase with age. When discussing cancer, or tumors, in this chapter, we will be referring to carcinomas. As well as carcinomas and sarcomas, there is another type of cancer that arises from immature white or red blood cells, known as leukemias.

Tumors contain outlaw cells! All other cells in our bodies have to obey certain rules about growth. Cancer cells ignore these rules of reproduction. Cancer cells are an example of what happens, when one tissue decides to look out for No. 1, and ignore the common good. Normally our stomach cells replace those lost from the abrasive action of foods, and the toxic and corrosive action of some chemicals, which we might swallow, but once these cells have been replaced, the reproduction stops. If it did not, we would all have stomachs as big as watermelons. Some people, unlucky enough to have gastric cancer, do have them.

Let's look at the behavior of law-abiding epithelial cells. Epithelium (plural form- epithelia) lines the body surfaces-external and internal body cavities. The skin, the linings of the air passages, and of the urogenital systems are all examples of epithelia. The epithelial cells of the skin, the gut, and the cervix renew themselves continually. Cells move towards the surface as they mature, being pushed that way by the continual production of new cells below them. The source of these new cells are stem cells, which themselves sit on a basement membrane. During this progression the cell goes through its life cycle, and upon reaching the upper surface, they are old. They remain on the surface for a time, and are then shed to the outside and sloughed off by the abrasion of food in the gut or other abrasive and mechanical forces, being replaced by cells migrating from the basement layer. So how does this well ordered process get upset?

Let's first get our names right! The new cells that the stem cells produce are daughter cells. The system that keeps our cellular reproduction under control has its root in the behavior of the stem cells. A stem cell divides to produce two cells. One daughter cell will go on to further reproduction; the other is destined to die without reproduction. A childless aunt, I suppose. The reproducing daughter cell will remain as a stem cell, while the maiden aunt will migrate to the surface to replace cells lost to attrition, and of course, will itself ultimately be lost the same way. So our epithelial tissues are kept in good order because of all of these childless aunts, selflessly giving up their rights to reproduce, and ultimately sacrificing themselves at the business end of the epithelium.

If, for some extraordinary reason, the reproduction from the stem cells were increased, this would usually be compensated for by a corresponding increase in the number of cells being lost at the surface. In this way the numbers of cells are kept pretty much the same most of the time. For there to be a fundamental loss of control, and that is what cancer is, something very unusual takes place: either more than 50 percent of the daughter cells would become reproductively capable stem cells; this means that the maiden aunts would have to indulge in illegal reproduction, or, some of the daughter cells covet immortality and continue to divide indefinitely. When this happens we get a movement towards carcinoma-a process called carcinogenesis.

Why do otherwise sensible cells suddenly become perverse in this way? Why do our maiden aunts suddenly dream of children of their own? Or why do some of the stem cells suddenly decide that they want to live forever? The cause is a failure in our system software. It is our software, the code in our DNA, which has within it an algorithm that governs reproduction, and the limits to it. When this code is damaged, the fail-safe inbuilt systems don't work. It is the system software, and only it, which tells the maiden aunts that the must simply live and die without reproducing (terminal differentiation), and that tells the daughter cells that they have to die and be discarded. When the system software fails, the system gets lawless!

Is this software anomaly hard to bring about? Not really! This aberrant reproductive behavior from cells can occur from a change in a relatively small set of genes. It is no wonder that cancer is so common. But there are repair systems, whose job it is to fix DNA-bugs. Debuggers, if you will.

The way in which cells reproduce (proliferate) is governed by a cell-cycle control system of protein switches. These proteins were developed by our ancestors about one billion years ago-oldies but goodies. They are present in almost every cell. You could take some of these old proteins from a yeast cell implant them into a human cell and they would work perfectly well.

As a cell enters the cell-division cycle, it produces proteins, which govern the whole operation. Each protein at each point in the cycle triggers the next protein, like dominos falling on each other. At particular points in this cycle however, the brakes are applied, while the cell checks that what is going on downstream, at the level of the cell substance, is coordinated with what is going on upstream, at the level of the nuclear system software. It is a system of falling dominoes with an intermittent feedback control system. At these checkpoints in the cycle, the whole system is regulated. This arrangement would bring a glow to the heart of any electrical engineer. This Universe is pretty darn smart! But of course, it was all an accident, wasn't it? Ha ha!

It is not only internal considerations that can arrest the process of cell division at these checkpoints. The cycle of division is sensitive to environmental signals that may at any point in the cycle shut it down. If external circumstances are not conducive to cell division a signal is received at checkpoint G1 (in mammalian systems), and cell division stops.

These protein-based cell-cycle feedback systems originate from DNA code in the genes. It is clear that when the DNA and therefore the genes has been damaged, that the feedback control system that governs cell division might not work in the usual way. DNA damage is common, so our cells have developed a feedback control system that operates in that event. Another protein, called p53, accumulates in the cell in response to DNA damage, and halts the cell cycle at checkpoint G1.

Mutations in the p53 gene play a vital role in the initiation of a large number of human cancers. When such a mutation occurs, the vital feedback control, which is meant to prevent DNA errors from being perpetuated into succeeding generations, is disabled. It is then that errors proliferate; cell division feedback controls are disabled, and an orgy of cell division ensues.

Around 1016 (10,000,000,000,000,000 or 10 quintillion) cell divisions take place in the human body during a lifetime. You do not need to have chemicals capable of producing mutations (mutagens) to get mutations. Mutations will happen spontaneously, even without mutagens. Even if you were able to live in an environment that was absolutely free of mutagens, and of course that is impossible, it is likely that during the course of a lifetime every single gene would have undergone a mutation on about 1,010 (10 trillion) separate occasions.

Of these many mutations, a large number could be expected to have occurred in genes that regulate cell division and proliferation. So it is surprising that cancer does not occur even more frequently.

Ten quintillion cell divisions in the course of an average lifetime mean that DNA has to copy itself ten quintillion times. With errors occurring every so often, it is clear that as we age there will be a greater and greater accumulation of errors. Because the chances of getting a genetic mutation increases as we age, so too do our chances of acquiring most cancers increase. Indeed, cancer incidence increases with age quite steeply.

Of course, there are some agents in our environment that can significantly increase our chances of having the type of genetic mutation that is likely to lead to cancer. These are called mutagens, or carcinogens, and we have known about them for a long time. Seventy percent of all cancers in humans arise from environmental factors, and more than 1,000 different chemicals have been identified as being cancer-producing.

If given the number of cell divisions that take place, it is easy to make copying errors in all of those trillions, quadrillions, and quintillions of cell divisions, why don't mutations occur more often? Our DNA has a built in proofreader whose job is to look at copied DNA strands and check them for errors.

We now know much more about cancer than any other generation. We know that it consists of a large group of diseases and is characterized by anomalous changes in cells, which can be transmitted to daughter cells. We know these changes originate from mutations in DNA. We know a wide range of stimuli can trigger such a mutation, including physical, chemical, and viral agents.

We know cancer is usually precipitated after a long exposure to such carcinogenic stimuli, and that it can be influenced by many environmental factors, including nutrition, genetics, and immune status. So although ancient, cancer is in many ways, a disease for our time.

There are a several reasons for this. Firstly, cancer is, for the most part, a disease of old age. There are such things as childhood and even infant cancers but most cancer results from changes in cell genetics, which progress into cancerous abnormalities over a longer period of time.

Most people throughout history, and even into modern times, have died from some other cause, before their body has had the time to generate cancer. This is less so for our generation. Ours is the first, for which old age is a general expectation. The second reason why cancer is a contemporary disease is because of better diagnosis today. There were probably many people in the past who had cancer, but whose cause of death was attributed to something else. With modern pathology, cancer is more often detected than not, and often at an early stage, when treatment has a better chance of success.

Why does cancer usually take so long to develop? It starts from one abnormal cell, a mutant ancestor-cell. This gives rise through many cycles of mutation and natural selection to a population of slightly abnormal cells. The development of the disease depends to a large degree on chance occurrences, and a lot of time. For cancer to occur there must be two processes going on- two series of events and/or agents. Those events and agents that cause cancer, the initiators, and those events and agents that speed up its development, the promoters. We will now look at how these factors are said to work together looking at skin cancer, as an example.

If a population of cells is subjected to continuous and serious genetic damage, say from serious and continuing exposure to radiation, or to a carcinogenic chemical, the chances are higher that enough cells will be genetically altered in a way likely to produce a cancerous tissue. The more cells affected, the more likely the abnormal behavior will be perpetuated. This first factor that causes the cells to become abnormal is called the initiator. After the abnormality has been established, it then needs other factors working for it to help it along. These other factors are tumor promoters. For cancer to be successful it needs one or more initiators, and one or more promoters.

It has been known for some time that coal tar is carcinogenic. In 1775 Percival Potts published a landmark article, in which he named many chemical carcinogens. One was coal tar.

There is a chemical in coal tar that causes cancer. It is also in tobacco smoke. These agents are initiators. They cause genetic damage and lead to a situation where a serious irritation, or repeated exposure to the initiator, or exposure to some other agent, will lead to cancer.

These latter substances are called promoters. Tumor promoters are common. We are encountering them all the time. But a tumor promoter will not cause cancer on its own, nor will a tumor initiator, but when you put the two together in the correct order cancer is likely.

In cancer of the skin, for example, it seems to be the initiator causes the genetic damage, and this can be latent (and harmless) for many years, until the tumor promoter comes along, and stimulates cell division in these abnormal cells. Such stimulation causes the growth of small, benign, wart-like tumors, called papillomas, on the skin. Because it is the initiator that causes the mutation, and the promoter which is responsible for the subsequent growth, the greater the exposure to the initiator, the more the number of papillomas.

A typical papilloma may contain 100,000 cells. As continued exposure to the promoter is required for growth of the abnormal cells, almost all papillomas will regress, if this exposure is stopped. Both wounding, and the application of the promoter, is likely to cause the tumor to develop, because both events favor cell division.

Because cancer is such a complicated, multi-step process, it is not easy to get. Many factors need to be working together for it to be successful. These include the genetic constitution of the individual and certain environmental circumstances. You can therefore drastically reduce your chances of contracting cancer by adopting certain lifestyle practices, and by avoiding others.

This can be strikingly shown by epidemiology, a science launched in 1713 by Bernadino Ramazzini of Padua, Italy. This scientist noticed that breast cancer occurred more frequently among Roman Catholic nuns than in the female population at large. This observation was followed a little later by the one from Potts on chimney sweeps. From such epidemiological observations we have learned a great deal about possible initiators and promoters of cancer. Cancer of the nose among the users of snuff was reported by John Hill in 1761. In 1895 Hartig reported high rates of bronchogenic carcinoma among miners in the Black Forest of Germany. In 1915 Yamagiwa and Ichikawa reported the carcinogenic effect of coal tar on rabbit skin. In the 1940s, researchers noted higher rates of uterine cancer among women of lower economic status, those who had early first sexual experience, and those who had multiple sexual partners. The association between lung cancer and cigarette smoking was suspected clinically in 1950, and later proven in controlled studies. All of these studies have done an enormous amount to help us understand what it is that certain people are doing which predisposes them to cancer.

Epidemiologists are still making these important and painstaking observations, with some striking results. For every country with a very high incidence of a particular cancer, there is another where the incidence of that particular cancer is very low.

For example, lung cancer is high in the USA among New Orleans African Americans, but low in Madras India. Breast cancer is high among Polynesian Hawaiians but low amongst Israeli non-Jews. Prostate cancer is high among African Americans in Atlanta, but low in Tianjin China. Cervical cancer is high in Recife Brazil but low in Israel. Stomach cancer is high in Nagasaki Japan, but low in Kuwait amongst the native Kuwaitis, and so it goes on. For every type of cancer reported by The International Agency for Research on Cancer in its 1997 report titled Cancer on Five Continents, there is a location where the incidence is high and another where it is quite low. This suggests that to a large degree, cancer is influenced by environmental factors.

Observations such as these suggest that 80 to 90 percent of cancer should be avoidable. The problem is that different cancers have different risk factors, and although you may be able avoid one, it is not always easy to avoid them all. For this reason, although cancer rates for a particular cancer varies from country to country, the overall cancer rate (at a given age) is similar between countries. But, there are some isolated and abstemious populations around the world, like the Mormons of Utah, who have very low incidence rates of all cancers.

What is intriguing about this epidemiological data, is trying to tease out what factors amongst the infinite variety available, are responsible for this variation in incidences. Take for example, the striking observation of Bernardino Ramazzini of Padua, the man who was, as we have seen, the first scientific epidemiologist. In 1713 he found that breast cancer occurred more often among Roman Catholic nuns than in the female population at large. This observation was confirmed by Domenico Rigoni-Stern in 1844. What could it be that was causing this? Burning candle wax? Incense? Small bread wafers? An act of God? Hardly!

Early observations, such as these, had to wait for others, before it was realized what was likely to be causing this effect. One such observation was that of Stevenson, who in 1913 observed that breast cancer rates were markedly higher after the age of 45 in single women than in married women. Then, in 1926, Lane-Claypon demonstrated a correlation between breast cancer among women who had never had children, or who had borne their first child at a later age. What was it, that all of these situations had in common? All of these individuals, the nuns and other single women, the childless and late-bearing women, all had one thing in common: high levels of the hormone estrogen for much of their reproductive lives. Might then, they asked, the hormone estrogen be a promoter of breast cancer?

This suggestion of a cause needed other confirming data. It was available, but for a long time no one noticed. One of the first to provide this was George Beatson of Glasgow, who reported in 1896 that pre-menopausal women who formerly had a spreading breast cancer had experienced tumor regression after removal of their ovaries (oophorectomy). This was later confirmed by H. Lett in 1905. Unfortunately, these early and important observations were essentially ignored for most of the 20th century, only to be rediscovered in 1950s when endocrine therapy was understood and used to achieve tumor regression in pre-menopausal women.

Cancer is characterized by a disruption of the normal restraints on cell division and proliferation. Control over cell division is the role of genes. Of the genes, which govern cell division, there are basically two types; those that stimulate reproduction, and those that inhibit it. When genes mutate so as to produce uncontrolled cell division (cancer), they can do so in two ways. The first of these occurs if the gene that stimulates cell reproduction becomes overactive. In such a case, the mutated gene is called an oncogene (from the Greek word ogkos meaning mass). It is a dominant gene. It can exert its influence, whether or not, the other member of the gene pair is similar to it. Genes occur in pairs, and each pair has a particular position on the chromosome.

The second progression to the disease occurs if the mutation causes the gene that suppresses cell division to become inactive (inhibits it). A gene that suppresses reproduction is recessive. It tends not to exert its influence, unless it pairs with a similar gene.

The abnormality in cell division, which we call cancer, can be aided by contact with certain chemicals, acting either as an initiator or promoter, such as cigarette smoke.

Other agents known to cause cancers are some viruses. A virus was discovered as a cause of cancer in chickens 80 years ago. This was the Rous sarcoma virus, a retrovirus. When a retrovirus infects a cell, the viral RNA is copied into the infected cell's DNA. Normally it is the other way around, with DNA giving rise to RNA. This is why they are called retroviruses, retro being the Latin word for backwards. If you add a tumor virus to a culture of normal cells you will soon get small colonies of transformed cells, each colony being derived from a single cell that has incorporated the genetic material from the virus.

These transformed cells proliferate madly, and pile up in layers. They have an altered shape, and they do not adhere to surfaces in the way that normal cells do. They do this because the retrovirus inserts an oncogene into the DNA of the host. This gene, which has been named src in the Rous sarcoma virus, is responsible for the cell transformation.

Scientists have isolated and sequenced (worked out the structure of) the src gene from the Rous sarcoma virus and found that it closely resembles a sequence found in the DNA of normal vertebrate cells. This sequence, which in the normal cells is called c-src, or just src, is identical to the sequence found in the virus, v-src. The c-src sequence found in normal cells seems to be a proto (a precursor) oncogene.

It seems that the virus picked up and cloned this sequence from humans, or some other vertebrate host, and it has been part of the viral genetic repertoire ever since. Many other oncogenes have now been recognized in other retroviruses, and for each one it has been found that there is a corresponding proto-oncogene in every normal cell.

About 60 proto-oncogenes have been discovered. Each one of these can, under the right circumstances, be converted into an oncogene.

What is the role of the proto-oncogenes in the normal cell? Are they just booby-traps inserted into our DNA by some malevolent deity? Or do they actually serve some higher purpose? It seems that most of the proto-oncogenes do have a role, to regulate the social behavior of the cell. They are particularly involved in the messages that cells get from their neighbors that cause them to divide, differentiate, or die. This is cell signaling. It is the way that cells talk to each other, and most of the proteins for this very important capacity of cells are coded for by proto-oncogenes.

It seems that if the proto-oncogene is altered by contact with a carcinogen or a virus, it begins to code for much more cell division than is needed. So the genetic basis of cancer, so far as it is understood, seems to be an important normal function, which goes awry. A genetic accident turns these useful proto-oncogenes into dangerous oncogenes.

What kind of genetic accident is necessary? As we have seen, the progression into a cancerous state does not depend on a single mutation in a single gene. Experiments on transgenic mice seem to suggest that what is needed to produce cancer is the synergistic collaboration between two or more oncogenes, a process known as oncogene collab-oration. The necessity in cancer for abnormalities to come from several directions at the same time relates back to the brilliant control systems built into our bodies by evolution. These fail-safe controls are only over-whelmed when they are assaulted from a number of directions at the same time. A single faulty component is not enough to bring the whole system crashing down.

We have a highly complex interaction of proto-oncogenes and tumor suppresser genes. The suppresser genes, most of the time, are pre-venting the transformation of a cell to a cancerous state. It is usually only when we, through infection, or other environmental factors, shift the balance toward the activation of the oncogene, or the inhibition of the suppresser gene that a serious disease begins to develop.

Viruses can be the trigger, and indeed in 15 percent of human can-cers they are. Examples are papilloma virus and cervical cancer, hepati-tis B virus and hepatocellular (liver) cancer, Epstein-Barr virus and Burkitt's lymphoma, HIV and Kaposi's sarcoma. Mostly in humans, unlike animals, it is DNA viruses, not retroviruses, which appear to be the culprits.

The connection between cancers and certain viruses have been detected in cancer patients. Certain forms of cancer are more prevalent in regions, which have a higher incidence of a particular virus. For example, liver cancer is more common in areas of the world where hep-atitis-B is also more common, and in those areas it tends to occur in suf-ferers from this disease.

Viruses have their effect in different ways. With hepatitis B, it seems that the virus first does damage to the liver, provoking cell division, and that this cell division can in the presence of the virus, get out of con-trol. In some other cancers, the viruses directly cause the transformation of the infected cells into cancer cells by altering their genes.

Such a genetic transformation must be a stable one, which can be propagated from generation to generation. This occurs by the host cell incorporating the viral DNA into its own chromosomes, and so creat-ing an oncogene. This type of genetic interference by viruses occurs from both DNA and retroviruses. DNA viruses, such as papilloma viruses, the cause of human warts, are also implicated in cancer of the cervix, and are able to take over the host's DNA synthesis machinery. Viruses, which can do this, can themselves act as oncogenes. Once the infection has taken place, the genes of the papilloma virus produce proteins, which inactivate two of the host's tumor-suppresser genes.

One of the tumor-suppresser genes that viruses tend to inactivate is *p53*. People who inherit only one functional copy of the *p53* suppresser gene (instead of two) have a genetic predisposition to develop cancer. People with this inherited deficiency in the *p53* gene are victims of the Li-Fraumeni syndrome. Fortunately quite rare, it predisposes them to a number of cancers, usually in early adulthood. The usual role of the *p53* is to produce a protein, which stops cells from dividing under hostile conditions, such as high levels of radiation, or other environmental factors, likely to cause DNA damage. The *p53* protein is part of the negative feedback loop on cell division, so that loss or inactivation of it removes an important block against uncontrolled cell division. Mutations of the *p53* gene accounts for more than 50 percent of all cancers.

Cancer, most commonly, is not a disease that suddenly appears, but is a disease that develops slowly, often the result of series of accidents or irritation.

Colorectal cancers are the second highest cause of cancer deaths in the US, and the figures are similar for Australia, UK, and other Western industrialized countries. Colo-rectal cancers are cancers of the cells lining the colon and rectum. Many aging people have small benign tumors in their colon. These are called *adenomatous polyps, or adenomas.* They could be precursors of malignant disease if left untreated, but if all people over the age of 55 have a colonoscopy every couple of years there should not be a problem from this disease.

Another thing that you can do to prevent colorectal cancer is to make sure that you get adequate dietary fiber. Bacteria in the colon love fiber. They convert it to short-chain fatty acids (SCFAs), such as acetic, proprionic, and butyric acids. These SCFAs are fuel for the cells lining the colon. They also tend to shrink the existing polyps, and prevent the formation of new ones. Butyrate, in particular, has been shown to cause malignant and pre-malignant cells in the colon to commit suicide (programmed cell death or apoptosis). Americans could reduce the incidence of colon cancer by approximately 31 percent, if fiber intakes from food sources were increased by about 13 g a day. This is the amount of fiber in an average-sized apple, or half a cup of cooked legumes.

Let's now look at fiber. Fiber is present in many vegetables and cereals. Pears, bananas, onions, and most of the cruciferous vegetables are high in it. Fiber forms the structural elements of plants, and is in the leaves, stems, roots, and fruit. For it to be of benefit in the prevention of colonic cancer, it has to be able to reach the colon. For most of the insoluble fibers, such as wheat bran, this is not a problem, because it is relatively indigestible in the higher gut. Insoluble fiber is a polysaccharide, which can be broken down by our colonic bacteria when it gets to the colon.

Starch is also a polysaccharide and a form of stored energy for the plant. Plants, like us, obtain their energy by oxidizing glucose. We obtain our glucose from plants, and they make their glucose by photosynthesis. This is the process by which plants synthesize glucose from CO_2, H_2O, and sunlight. If plants could not store their glucose, they would starve during the night, when the sun was not available. Similarly, we store our glucose in a molecule called glycogen, which itself is stored in the liver, and in muscles.

For starch to be of use in the prevention of colonic cancer, it must be amylase-resistant. It has to avoid being digested and absorbed higher up the gastrointestinal tract. Our saliva and our pancreatic secretions contain an enzyme, amylase, which breaks down starch so that it can be absorbed in the small intestine.

Which fibers are amylase-resistant? Wheat bran reaches the colon, where it is partially digested by the colonic bacteria. A bolus containing insoluble fiber such as this acts like a giant broom, sweeping the colonic contents (with bile salts bound to toxins) out of the colon. As an incidental benefit, your blood cholesterol falls, because you are excreting cholesterol in bile salts. Often when starch such as that found in potato or rice is cooled after cooking, it undergoes a chemical change, a polymerization reaction that makes it amylase-resistant. So, cooled cooked potato and rice supply resistant starch.

Oligosaccharides are short-chain sugars in edible plants, such as chicory, onion, artichoke, and soybeans. These vegetables have non-digestible oligosaccharides, which stimulate the growth of colonic LAB. Resistant starches and certain non-soluble fibers do reach the colon, where the colonic bacteria ferment them. There are even commercial breads available that claim to contain resistant starch.

In addition to looking at your starch and fiber intake, it is, of course, important to make sure that your levels of good bacteria remain high. There are more than 400 different bacterial species in the gut. Bacteria account for 35 to 50 percent of the colon contents by volume. The levels of these colonic bacteria fluctuate in response to many environmental factors, including antibiotics, alcohol, and stress, so in order to keep your colon healthy, it may be necessary to take LAB. Lactobacillus acidophilus and lactobacillus bifido are contained in many available yogurts.

Another useful LAB is lactobacillus casei. These LAB, not only give us a healthy colon, but also stimulate our immune system generally, and make it harder for pathogenic bacteria and yeasts to get a foothold. In addition, they suppress the activity of harmful enzymes such as beta-glucuronidase, nitro-reductase, and azoreductase, and enhance the desirable enzymes, such as beta-galactosidase, which is useful in the alleviation of lactose intolerance.

These LAB do not always stay in the gut, but enter the general circulation. Lactobacilli can travel, or translocate, and can survive many days in the spleen, liver and lungs. During their travels they can stimulate the immune system locally, by enhancing the activity of phagocytes, natural killer cells, and have a role in the prevention of tumor growth.

Dietary saturated fats, not only play a significant role in the development of heart disease, but contribute as well to a number of cancers, including colorectal cancer. They are therefore best avoided.

When you do have fats, take instead the monounsaturated variety, such as those in olive and canola oils, as well as the important desaturated essential FAs found in evening primrose oil and fish. Too much sunflower and safflower oil contains LA and this FA is not particularly good for us, since most of us cannot desaturate it.

If at risk of colorectal cancer, you should be assiduous about reducing your SaFA consumption. As well, it may be efficacious to increase your intake of calcium. Studies have shown that a good intake of dietary calcium, about 1200 mg a day protects against colorectal cancer.

Calcium may be protective because it binds the FAs and bile salts to form a soap that washes the fat out of our gut. A dose of 1200mg is about twice the calcium in the usual consumption Western diet.

It is also important to make sure that you have adequate antioxidants, principally vitamin E and beta-carotene, for two reasons. Firstly, the colonic bacteria themselves produce ROS, such as the superoxide ion, and secondly, vitamin E will prevent the fats in the colon forming the harmful and carcinogenic oxidation products and mutagens.

The other lifestyle and dietary factors that increase the risk of this disease are low folate, high alcohol consumption, and cigarette smoking.

Those at risk of the disease, such as those with a family history of it, should be very careful about alcohol consumption. Each alcoholic drink (especially beer and spirits) consumed a day was found by one group to increase the risk of colon cancer by 17 percent, with the risk being even higher in smokers.

Communities, which have high intakes of red meat also have high levels of colonic cancer. Red meat and preserved meats have high levels of chemicals called nitrates and nitrites. These are converted to N-nitrosamine in the gut after consumption, which is thought to exert a carcinogenic effect on the colon and in stomach.

These N-nitroso compounds have been measured in feces, and found to be higher in those who consumed high levels of red meat. Chicken and fish consumption does not have this association with N-nitroso compounds.

One of the best ways to help prevent colon cancer is to eat lots of cruciferous (so called because the petals of their flowers form a cross) vegetables, preferably uncooked. These include, cabbage, Brussels sprouts, cauliflower, and broccoli. They are high in dietary fiber, glutathione, and sulfur-containing compounds (thiols), all of which have been found to be useful in helping to prevent colorectal cancer. They are also helpful as a breast cancer preventative.

Cruciferous vegetables seem to stimulate the liver's cytochrome P450 detoxification pathway, as does an herb called St. Mary's thistle or silymarin. So that the liver is better able to chemically change, and render soluble, many of the genotoxic (poisonous to our genes) substances, which we commonly encounter in the 21st century. The P450 detoxification pathway operates by means of cytochrome reactions, in a similar way to the ETC of the mitochondria, and so is subjected to oxidant damage, in the same way. As a consequence our detox pathway becomes less efficient with aging, as this oxidant stress takes its toll.

So the daily consumption of these cruciferous vegetables is one of the secrets of good health. Silymarin is considered by many who should know, like professional wine-tasters, as an excellent hangover preventative. That would make sense, because it enhances the liver's ability to detoxify this chemical.

Breast cancer is the most common cancer among women in industrialized countries, and the second most common in non-industrialized ones. About one American woman in 11 will develop breast cancer. It is sometimes seen in women in their twenties, but is not common until after the age of 40. A more usual age is around 60.

The type of breast cancer to which I refer is the estrogen-positive form of the disease.

Family history, whether or not your mother or sister has the disease, is an important risk factor, accounting for an almost fivefold increase in risk. The risk factor that seems most to predispose women to breast cancer however is the length of time that the breast tissue has been exposed to the hormone estrogen.

From the beginning of menstrual bleeding to menopause, substantial amounts of the hormones estrogen and progesterone are produced by the ovary, and in particular, by the corpus luteum of the ovarian follicle.

These hormones cause an increase in proliferation (growth) of breast tissue. It is these surges of growth-inducing hormones, such as estrogen that are primarily responsible for breast cancer. After menopause, when most people suffer from the disease, it is true that these surges have stopped, but by the time that happens, the damage has already been done.

At the risk of sounding like an ultra-right wing conservative, the ideal way for a woman to avoid breast cancer is for her to be continuously either pregnant or lactating all of her reproductive life. Carrying and nursing babies, and especially having the first baby early in life, puts a brake on the effects of the hormone estrogen.

A pregnant woman is subject to enormous hormone surges, including the hormone estrogen, but has special protection, in the form of a special protein, called the fetal steroid binding protein.

This protein binds to the estrogen receptors in the breast tissue of the pregnant woman, and prevents estrogen from so binding. In this way, pregnancy gives protection from breast cancer. If a woman has a baby early in her reproductive life she gets this protection. If she delays childbearing, as women frequently choose to do in Western societies, the estrogen-based damage might have already been done by the time she has the child. In choosing to delay childbearing, she has lost her opportunity for protection.

Breast-feeding decreases the risk of breast cancer because it too decreases the exposure of the breast tissue to estrogen. After a baby is born, the concentrations of estrogen and progesterone fall, as these hormones would inhibit milk production, if at their pre-birth levels. After birth, another hormone, prolactin, increases and stimulates milk production. Breast-feeding puts the brakes on estrogen.

There are some other risk factors apart from estrogen to consider. Oral contraceptives are responsible for a small increase in the risk of breast-cancer, but usually this is only during the time that the medication is being taken. Fat and alcohol consumption is a significant risk factor for both breast cancer and colon cancer.

Another important risk factor is obesity. Because fat cells produce estrogen, obese women have a supply of this hormone, which slim women don't have.

Strategies for the prevention of breast cancer therefore would include, weight loss, reducing alcohol and fat intake, increasing exercise, and the consumption of fresh fruit and vegetables. Vegetables are a preventative against all cancer, because they provide antioxidants.

There is one other helpful preventative of breast cancer, phytoestrogens. Both men and women produce male and female sex hormones. Men produce the female hormone estrogen in very small quantities, and women the male hormone testosterone, also in very small quantities. Men get very much less breast cancer than women, because they produce large amounts of the hormone testosterone, which tends to block estrogen. Women do not get this protection.

Women however, and men too for that matter, can get the type of protection offered by testosterone by eating soy products, as well as foods made from legumes, and from linseed. These foods contain what is called phytoestrogens, naturally occurring substances with chemical similarities to estrogen made by plants. These bind to the estrogen receptor in the breast tissue, so preventing estrogen from doing this. Indeed, this is exactly how Tamoxifen® works.

Tamoxifen® is a synthetic drug used as a preventative for breast cancer. It has been known to have some unpleasant side effects in some women. Phytoestrogens are nature's Tamoxifen®. They are side effect free, and some say, at least as effective as the synthetic drug.

Japanese women have one-sixth the chance of American women of acquiring breast cancer. Many researchers think that the main reason for this is their consumption of soy products. The active ingredient in soy products is probably genistein. It seems that genistein, like Tamoxifen®, competes with estrogen for access to the estrogen receptor.

Physical exercise reduces breast-cancer risk. Perhaps it interferes with estrogen in some way. It is not uncommon, for example, for elite-athletic women to cease having periods (amenorrhoea). Even with moderate exercise, in one study involving adolescent girls it was found that exercise decreased ovulation. If ovulation is decreased, so is estrogen production, because the follicle of the ovary produces it.

The only other time amenorrhoea occurs is during pregnancy and lactation. These are also times when the estrogen has been interrupted.

It is said that fats are a significant risk factor for colorectal and breast cancer, but this is only part of the story. The proliferation of certain other types of cancer, that of the prostate, ovary, endometrium, pancreas, and bladder also seems enhanced by dietary fats.

There have been many laboratory studies over 40 years in which laboratory animals, mainly rats and mice, have been given 40 percent of their caloric intake in fat. This is a diet, which mimics the human diet in advanced countries, and it has been found to promote these cancers.

In these experiments however, the fats that were invariably used were SaFAs and t-FAs. Where PUFAs were used they tended to be the ones, which we consume the most of, such as LA. LA is a prominent FA found in seed oils, such as sunflower and safflower, and people eating large quantities of margarines made from these products, like Israelis, consume a lot of it. Not all polyunsaturated fats are good for us, and the evidence is quite strong that this is such a one. It does not have good effects when consumed in quantity. LA seems to stimulate the growth of cancer cells in the breast and other tissues, which are sensitive to FAs.

There is good evidence that saturated animal fats, and polyunsaturated vegetable oil fats (high in LA) can lead to increased tumor growth, but the evidence is equally strong that the desaturated essential FAs, such as those in evening primrose oil and fish, gamma linolenic acid (GLA), and eicosapentenoic acid (EPA) respectively, can stop the growth of, and even kill, certain cancer cells, under certain conditions.

The problem is then that, yes, consumption of fats is bad for you, in relation to CHD and the fat-sensitive cancers, but only certain types of fats, the ones which we in Western countries like to eat! In Australia, Western Europe, and North America, where fat comprises about 40 percent of the diet, the incidence of breast cancer is about 3-4 times higher than it is in Japan, where among those consuming a traditional diet large amounts of fish and rice are consumed. The traditional Japanese diet is not a low fat one, but rather one comparatively low in saturated fats and low in the particular N-6 PUFAs found in man-made margarines.

Although the consumption of phytoestrogens in soy products also helps to give some protection to Japanese women, the consumption of a large amount of fish in their diet is a big factor in their protection against breast cancer. There are other fish-eating populations who do not eat soy products, such as the Inuit people, who are also protected from fat-sensitive cancers by a diet high in fish oil.

The injection of both N-6 PUFAs found in evening primrose oil, and N-3 PUFAs from fish into breast tumors in rats reduces both the size and incidence of them.

Indeed, the increase in cancer that has occurred during much of the 20th century has coincided with the increased consumption of seed oil by humans and animals. During the 20th century, we have been increasingly feeding animals in unnatural ways, as well as ourselves using more processed food. This has had the overall tendency of reducing our consumption of unsaturated and desaturated FAs and replacing them with SaFAs and trans-isomers and LA. The period has also coincided with an increased consumption of meat in Western societies.

This modern sea change in dietary habits has also had a powerful effect on other chronic degenerative conditions, including atherosclerosis, CHD, pulmonary embolism, cerebrovascular disease, Chron's disease, diverticulosis, multiple sclerosis, osteoporosis, rheumatoid arthritis, nephrosis, renal stones, asthma, NIDDM, systematic lupus erythematosis, and certain viral diseases.

What I am referring to as desaturated FAs, include docosahexanoic acid (DHA), EPA and GLA. I call them desaturated because they have all undergone a desaturation reaction with an enzyme called delta-6-desaturase. We have this enzyme too, but, as we get older, and as a consequence of illness and other factors, it becomes inefficient. We can get around this biochemical block by taking DHA, EPA and GLA ready-made. In the first two the desaturase reaction has been undertaken by the marine animal, and in the last, it come to us, courtesy of a plant.

These fatty acids are not the only fats that might give some protection from fat-sensitive cancers, such as breast cancer. Another oil to be encouraged is olive oil. Breast cancer is less common like Italy and Greece, were the major fat consumed is from olive oil, than in USA,

UK and Australia. It is possible that something in the olive oil can inhibit the metabolic activation of carcinogens. It is therefore, not all fats that we must avoid, just saturated ones, trans-FAs and LA.

GLA, EPA and olive oil (oleic acid) are the good oils, the oils of gladness. They will not kill a cancer patient, but could kill his/or her cancer, particularly when combined with high doses of coenzyme Q_{10}.

What are the reasons for the apparently protective effect of the desaturated EFAs with cancer? David Horrobin, a pioneer in the use of GLA against cancer, has put forward the idea that cancer cells cannot tolerate GLA in the same way that normal cells can, and as a consequence, dosing on these FAs causes a destructive lipid peroxidation cascade to occur in the cancer cell.

The second idea about how these FAs can influence cancer is deduced from what we know about the way in which cancer spreads.

A cancer in an epithelial tissue, say, starts out as a single mutant cell. This develops into a colony of abnormal cells-a stage called dysplasia. The colony will grow and ultimately break through the basement membrane at its boundary if not arrested. It is in this way that epithelial cancers spread or metastasize, and this makes the cancer becomes very hard to treat.

A cancer which does not spread, a cancer in situ, can be treated by killing-off the affected cells, but once the cancer has metastasized, or become malignant, it can become very widely distributed seeding colonies of cancer cells in many locations.

The breaking away of the cancer, by breaking through a basement membrane, and the consequent carriage of the cancer cells into the blood and lymph vessels below this membrane, is very important to the survival of the cancer. How does cancer do this? How does it break through the basement membrane?

It has to degrade collagen in the basement membrane, by activating receptors, called protease receptors, on the membrane of the target cell. The cancer activates the protease receptors by secreting a chemical, a urokinase-type plasminogen activator (uPA). Once the protease receptors are activated, the cell secretes collagenase, which helps it to digest the extracellular material around it, including the basement membrane below it.

It is in this way that the cancer breaks out of its tissue cage, and travels to (invades) other tissues. GLA (from evening primrose oil) and EPA (from fish oil) are inhibitors of uPA. Treatment with GLA makes cancer cells less invasive. The inhibition of the uPA system by them could be why the FAs (desaturated ones) found in fish, and evening primrose oil, are an efficacious therapy for cancer treatment, especially when combined with Coenzyme Q_{10} .

Cancer of the cervix of the uterus is the leading cause of malignancy afflicting developing countries. Epidemiological evidence suggests that viruses passed into the cervix during sexual intercourse may be important in this disease. The chief suspect is Herpes virus hominis type 2 the genital herpes virus. Eighty percent of women with the tumor also test positive to this virus.

Sexual relations at an early age are also considered to be a risk factor, as is sexual intercourse with multiple partners. Nuns have a minimal risk of this disease (although have a high risk of breast cancer), and prostitutes have a very high risk. In countries where almost all the men are circumcised, there is little or no cervical cancer among the women. The cumulative incidence in Israel is less than 1 percent, while in Colombia it is nearly 7 percent.

The Pap (Papanicolaou) smear, a cheap and efficient screening test for this disease, has saved many lives. One researcher has calculated that failure to have the Pap smear over 5 years increases the clinical risk of invasive carcinoma by 5 times.

What can we do as a preventative for cervical cancer? High levels of glutathione have been found to help protect against it. It may be that the infectious agents that might initiate the disease might be responsible for the production of free radicals.

We know that phagocytes do produce free radicals in response to infection. It may be then that the cells of the uterine cervix are particularly sensitive to free radicals produced in this way, and become genetically abnormal as a result. If this is so, then it is no surprise that high levels of glutathione are found to be protective, since glutathione is a superb antioxidant.

Glutathione can be found in asparagus, watermelon, and avocados, but if I were at risk of cervical cancer I would be taking the reduced form of glutathione (GSH) as a supplement daily. In addition to cervical cancer, low levels of glutathione have also been associated with malignancies in the breast, lung, liver, prostate gland, and lymphoma.

One cancer that has responded to environmental changes is cancer of the stomach, or gastric cancer. In 1930, it was the leading cause of cancer mortality among men in the US. Since then the incidence of this cancer has been falling in Western countries possibly because of H. pylori has also declined. H. pylori were once common in Western countries, although still extensive in developing countries, and these countries have a high incidence of this disease.

A family history of the disease contributes to the risk of contracting it. If this disease runs in your family, you have 2 to 3-times a greater chance of contracting it. This is particularly the case, if blood type A also runs in the family.

Gastric cancer today, represents about 3 percent of all American cancer deaths, but it has a high incidence in countries such as Korea, Japan, and China, in the former USSR, Costa Rica, and South America. This strongly suggests that it is largely due to environmental factors.

Prominent among these additional environmental risk factors is N-nitrosamine, a carcinogen produced from dietary nitrates and nitrites. Bacteria in the gut and elsewhere accomplish this conversion.

Antioxidants can inhibit this transformation. N-nitrosamine, H. pylori, and salt, together and separately, disturb the gastric muscosa, resulting is chronic gastritis and atrophy. The intermediate stages of the transformation of a normal stomach cell into a cancer cell involve a change to even more extreme cellular abnormalities called metaplasia and dysplasia. The final cellular change is one to cancer.

This bleak procession may be interrupted, at least in the early stages, by antioxidants found in fruit and vegetables. Antioxidants such as beta-carotene and vitamins C and E prevent the conversion of nitrates/nitrites to N-nitrosamine, and therefore may help to protect against gastric cancer. People, who have low levels of beta-carotene, are at increased risk of gastric cancer risk. High plasma levels of beta-carotene, Se, and vitamin C are all associated low death rates form gastric cancer, as well as cancers of the esophagus.

Red and processed meats are a source of N-nitosamine, so are cigarettes. Even one cigarette a day increases the risk of gastric cancer by over four-times because of the N-nitrosamine which they contain.

A large Chinese population based study found that men, who smoked one or more packs of cigarettes a day, had a 50 percent greater gastric cancer risk than non-smokers. Similar results were obtained from a study in the US. The inhalation of the dusts of certain metals, such as beryllium, nickel and chromium, as well as that of cement and coal dust also increased the risk of gastric cancer.

Cigarettes, beer, Scotch, and whisky all contain pre-formed N-nitrosamines, the gastric carcinogens. In addition, alcohol itself may increase the risk of gastric cancer, as indicated by a French study, where red wine which does not contain nitrosamines was associated with gastric cancer, when consumed at levels above 19 oz. (half a liter) of alcohol per week.

High intakes of barbecued or smoked foods (more than twice a week) also are thought to increase gastric cancer risk, presumably because they are high in N-benzyl pyrene and/or nitrites. In Japan and Iceland, intakes of cured and smoked meats and fish are high and so are gastric cancer risks.

Preventative measures against gastric cancer include: lots of fruits and vegetables, moderation in alcohol, and reduced intake of smoked and salted foods. In countries where night soil is a fertilizer, care should be taken to prevent fecal and oral transmission of H. pylori.

Methionine has recently been found to be a risk factor for gastric cancer. It seems that nitrate, salt, and methionine together, produce a newly discovered mutagen, 2-chloro-4-methylthiobutanoic acid (CMA), which has been found in the nitrite-rich Japanese fish, Sanma hiraki. A northern Italian study found that a high dietary intake of methionine was associated with significant gastric cancer risk. People with high intakes of salt and methionine had nearly three times the risk. Red meat, itself associated with gastric cancer, is high in methionine and nitrates/nitrites.

Better handling of food, especially refrigeration, and the elimination of salting, as a means of preservation has been largely responsible for the universal decline in gastric cancer. The bacterial conversion of nitrates and nitrites has declined with the widespread use of refrigeration, and the consequent reduction in incidence of H. pylori. Refrigeration has also meant a wider availability of fruit and vegetables, and a decline in the conversion of dietary nitrates/nitrites to the carcinogenic N-nitroso compounds.

In the United States, primary lung cancer represents about 15 percent of all cancer cases (22 percent in males and 8 percent in females). The disease causes 25 percent of all cancer deaths. The predominant risk factor is cigarette smoking, with a contribution made from exposure to industrial chemicals.

English physician John Hill first reported a relationship between tobacco use and carcinoma in 1761, but the first modern paper linking cigarette smoking and cancer was not published until 1950. Since then, all credible studies, prospective and retrospective, have consistently shown a strong statistical relationship between smoking and lung cancer. The mortality rate from lung cancer among male cigarette smokers is approximately eight to fifteen times that of those who never smoked.

Until recently, the scientific and medical community was fairly unanimous about the fact that cigarette smoking contributed so much to lung cancer that it could be considered, pretty much the sole cause. Recently, that opinion has come under some review. The American Journal of Respiration in its edition of February 1999, reported on a 16-year study of more than 6000 non-smokers in California, which found a significant association between levels of airborne particles, and the number of deaths from lung cancer in males. A strong link was also found, between O_3 levels and lung cancer in men, and sulfur dioxide and lung cancer in both men and women. O_3 and sulfur dioxide are generated as a consequence of the effects of sunlight on vehicle exhausts, photochemical smog, as well as exhaust from other industrial processes.

The fact that males are more at risk than females is interesting, and it shows up in many studies. Probably it reflects the fact, that men are usually outdoors more than women. So there is more to it than simply looking at smoking.

Lung cancer has also been associated with certain industrial chemicals, including asbestos, radon amongst uranium workers, and zeolite fibbers, but cigarette smoking is the principal cause of this disease. Not only is it a risk for lung cancer, but also for cancers in the following sites: lip, mouth, tongue, larynx, esophagus, bladder, and pancreas. This makes cigarette smoke a general carcinogen, as well as a specific one for lung cancer. It joins a long list of other carcinogens in our environment.

A certain amount of protection against many of these chemical carcinogens has been shown by many studies to be provided by flavones; the antioxidant products in fruits and vegetables. Examples are quercetin found in onions and apples, and the indoles found in cruciferous vegetables. These chemicals inhibit the effects of a number of chemical carcinogens, including benzo[a] pyrene, a polycyclic aromatic hydrocarbon. Se salts are also protective.

We have seen earlier that free radicals and in particular the superoxide ion may be contributors to the cancer cascade. We also know that certain phagocytes produce the superoxide ion in their respiratory bursts, common in inflammation. So could it be possible that inflammation, that normal reaction of the body to infection and injury, is itself a promoter of cancer?

There is some evidence to support this notion, and it has been strengthened by experimental data. For example, Witz and her colleagues have found that with chemical tumor promoters, that the degree of superoxide ion generation is correlated with the degree of tumor promotion.

Others have established that the intake of transition metals, such as iron, which we know will facilitate the production of ROS through the Fenton reaction, is correlated with cancer development in humans and animals. Not only that, but we have known for some time that free radical-scavenging vitamins such as vitamins C and E can protect against cancer development. The cancer protective effect of these antioxidant vitamins is clear from animal experiments, and results have suggested that they may be protective to humans as well. The process of inflammation is similar for all mammals.

We saw that certain metals, such as nickel and chromium, are carcinogenic and this may at least in part, be due to their catalytic effect on oxidant reactions. We also know that chronic inflammatory states are also associated with the development of human malignancies. In addition, many of the chemical carcinogens we have just been discussing are known to do their damage via oxidant mechanisms.

Let's look at how inflammation and oxidant stress might have this effect. Mottram, Barenblum, and Shubik in the 1940s determined cancer to be a multistage process. They did most of their work on mouse skin. Since these epoch-making experiments, the multistage nature of cancer has been demonstrated in many other tissues, including, stomach, liver, pancreas, bladder, colon, lung, trachea, thyroid, and breast. Scientists now believe there are three stages to cancer, not two as the earlier researchers believed.

The first is initiation, where a single cell undergoes heritable mutation. This mutation is to genes that regulate growth and differentiation.

The second stage is the promotion, after exposure to a promoter, initiated cells are stimulated to grow-to make many more copies of themselves. This is clonal expansion. After this stage a tumor has begun, but it is still a benign tumor until it reaches the third stage, malignant conversion. This also requires genetic alteration, after which all growth is deregulated. Rafferty's Rules prevails, pretty much like capitalism in the late 20th and early 21st Centuries.

For all of these stages to proceed, mutations to the genes are required. This involves altering the DNA, and can be accomplished by oxidant stress. O_2 in bacteria changing DNA was first demonstrated 30 years ago, and other agents which increase the amount of O_2 in biological systems including activated neutrophils, have since been shown to cause damage and alteration to human DNA.

Experiments have shown that if you take some of these ROS and put them into a Petri dish containing cultured cells, they can be transformed into a malignancy. We know that hydroxyl radical is the most dangerous to DNA, so if you place into the Petri dish, some metal chelators (chemicals which block the formation of hydroxyl radical), you can inhibit DNA damage, mutations, and malignant transformations, that otherwise would be caused. The same effect is produced if you put into the Petri dish, agents that use up the hydroxyl radicals. But if allowed to remain, the highly reactive hydroxyl radical will interact with many components of the DNA molecule, producing a lot of damage.

Some of the damage recorded in experiments to DNA by hydroxyl radical will include modifications to all bases, base-free sites, deletions, strand-breaks, DNA-protein cross-links, and chromosomal rearrangement.

As we saw earlier, DNA has systems to repair the odd mistake that is bound to happen in replication and transcription, but if the damage is sufficiently stubborn and persistent, these are overwhelmed. Many of the genetic alterations caused by oxidant stress will kill the cell, and this will present no problem for the organism at large. However, some DNA deletion or rearrangement may survive, and promote gene dysregulation in the descendant cells.

This can result in gene inactivation. If the inactivation is in a tumor-suppresser gene, the result may be the initiation of carcinogenesis. If a critical base pair is deleted from the tumor-suppresser gene, the gene is inactivated. This can easily happen in a situation of acute oxidant stress.

Oxidant stress can induce initiation also by changing the base pairs in ordinary somatic genes, turning them into oncogenes. A usual site for such alterations is at the guanine-cytosine (G-C) base pairings. We know experimentally that the most frequent site of a mutation in the ras family of oncogenes is at the G-C pairs in codons 12 and 13. Moreas and colleagues have shown that DNA has a tendency to form mutations at G-C sites when exposed to oxidant stress, and that such alterations can survive replication and repair systems.

Other laboratory experiments show that when such a G-C alteration occurs, that it can often do so in the very genes responsible for growth regulation, namely in the p53 and in the retinoblastoma tumor-suppresser genes.

Copper is bound to DNA at the G-C sites, where it helps to stabilize the complicated DNA architecture. Copper is a transition metal that often takes a catalytic role in oxidation reactions, so the presence of copper at such a critical site may expedite the damage in an oxidant environment. Much research demonstrates that oxidant stress plays a role in the later stages of carcinogenesis, so the case for a role for oxidant stress in carcinogenesis is very strong.

What is the evidence that antioxidants may prevent the development of cancer? There is much literature attesting that antioxidants, such as vitamin C, vitamin E, Se, flavonoid, phenols, and carotenoids, can be protective against carcinogenesis.

Some 200 or more studies have been published on the association between vegetable and fruit intake and cancer in the lung, oral cavity, esophagus, stomach, rectum, pancreas, bladder, breast, cervix, and ovary. This evidence suggests that the protective effect of fruits and vegetables is most convincing for epithelial cancers (e.g. lung, esophagus, gut), especially those of the respiratory tract, and less convincing for hormone-related cancers, such as breast cancer. Block summarizes much of the work on the effects of vitamin C in non-hormone based cancer prevention studies. She says that for oral, esophageal, gastric, and pancreatic cancer, the evidence that vitamin C may provide some protection is strong.

Evidence supports the role of carotenoids in the protection against lung cancer, although beta-carotene should not be used if the subject is a smoker.

Pancreatic cancer is the fifth most common cause of cancer mortality in the United Sates, and it is a disease that usually has a poor prognosis. Five out of five studies involving fruit and vegetables and pancreatic cancer reported by Block demonstrated a protective effect. In relation to stomach cancer, seven out of seven investigators showed a protective effect from vitamin C. Not surprisingly, consumption of fresh fruit and vegetables was found to be protective as well.

For cervical cancer, the evidence tends to suggest that it is those who have the lowest levels of vitamin C in their plasma who are most likely to acquire the disease. High plasma levels of beta-carotene also accorded protection. Low maternal vitamin C levels have been associated with a threefold increased risk of delivering a child with a brain tumor. There is data supporting the idea that vitamin E protects against a wide range of cancers, although clinical trials are needed to definitively answer the question. The Basel study was a large prospective study of 4858 males over two separate periods of three years. The conclusion was: "*Our results leave no doubt that low carotene status is associated with an increased risk for bronchus cancer and overall cancer death (p 268S).*"

The evidence favors the proposition that oxidant stress has a prominent role in the production of cancer. One of the most important sources of oxidant stress is inflammation, the process by which our body dons a fighting fettle when we are deemed to be in danger, due to tissue injury, and infection. This response is a juggernaut that not even the most virulent invading microbe is likely to be able to resist, but for this high-tech weapon we must pay a price-oxidant stress. The phagocytic cells that have been attracted to the area start to produce respiratory bursts of ROS. These bursts, though very effective in killing off the invading microbe also cause, what has become known in modern warfare, as collateral damage.

The free radicals and other ROS produced by our immune system are not laser-guided weapons, they are more like a blast from a shotgun, and some of our cells are also damaged or killed by the friendly fire.

As with other wars, the only consolation being that much, much, more damage is done to the enemy. This is the way that inflammation causes damage by means of oxidant stress. If such damage alters our genes, and we know that it can, then we have moved a step closer to the initiation of cancer.

It is estimated that the number of oxidant hits to our DNA is about 10 000 a cell a day. Mostly, the damage done to our DNA by ROS is removed continuously by our DNA repair systems. But a small amount of the damage escapes repair. As we age, there is more and more of this damaged DNA. This is why our risk of cancer rises with aging. After a lifetime of oxidant damage to our DNA, we have much more mutagenic potential than we did when young, it being increased with oxidant stress.

If after developing this mutagenic potential we then come into contact with a mutagenic chemical or radiation, the deleterious effect of the initiating event is amplified by our oxidant stress. Low but consistent levels of oxidant stress can stimulate cell division, and promote tumor growth. One of the effects of ROS is to cause cells to increase their levels of calcium. This is an important event that mediates the induction of proto-oncogenes. ROS have been shown also to be able to directly regulate the activity of a transcription factor (transcription is the process by which RNA, for protein synthesis, is made from DNA) in the rel oncogene family. Thus, with aging and inflammation, and the oxidant stress that inevitably accompanies it, there is produced in us all a potential for cancer promotion, and sometimes, though perhaps rarely, tumor initiation itself.

If oxidant stress caused by inflammation contributes to cancer, why do drugs that help reverse inflammation, such as aspirin, not cure cancer? Aspirin may not cure cancer, but it can certainly help. So far, much of the data about the protection afforded by aspirin (and its relatives) relates to cancer of the large bowel (colon cancer), and there is lot of it. There is data also about aspirin giving protection from other types of cancer. Cancer of the tongue, esophagus, pancreas, bladder, breast, liver, various sarcomas, as well as many transplantable tumors, have benefited from it.

The best evidence from studies on humans relates to protection from colon cancer, where there is a 40 to 50 percent lower risk of fatal colon cancer in people regularly using aspirin, compared with those who use none, in a prospective study of over 600,000 adults in the United States. Another large study (635,031 men and women) in the US, by Thun and colleagues, found that: "*Aspirin use was associated with reduced risk of fatal cancers of the esophagus, stomach, colon, and rectum. The decreased risk of digestive tract cancers was similar in men and women; it was stronger in those with the more frequent and prolonged use of aspirin, and it could not be attributed to other risk factors for these cancers (p1324)."*

These real-world studies are supported by many laboratory studies, where aspirin and its relatives, called non-steroidal anti-inflammatory drugs (NSAIDs), have been found to prevent cell growth and proliferation, tumor growth, tumor promotion, and metastasis, as well as to improve general immune response. There were also two large studies, the Leisure World study, and the Physicians Health Study trial, which could not find a relationship between consumption of aspirin and cancer.

Bearing in mind the fact that a daily aspirin therapy can also help in the avoidance of CHD, it might be smart to take aspirin each day. What dose of aspirin? The dosage for prevention of CHD is less than 100 mg a day; say one quarter of a standard 300 mg aspirin tablet, so that to help prevent cancer should be the same, because it uses the same mechanism, namely prostaglandins and the metabolites of Ar. A.

Even aspirin, however, should be taken under medical supervision. Aspirin and other NSAIDs have been used for decades in the treatment of arthritis, often in quite high doses. Sometimes, such treatment causes bleeding from the gut as a side effect. There is also a condition called Reyes syndrome, named after the Australian physician, Ralph Douglas Kenneth Reye, it is a severe childhood disorder following a virus infection, such as chicken pox, rubella, influenza, herpes simplex, or echovirus. A characteristic of it is hepatitis, a dangerous swelling of the brain, coma and/or death. This condition is strongly associated with the use of aspirin, and, as a consequence, aspirin is no longer routinely given to children.

Although an adult is unlikely to have any problems taking a daily dose of 75 mg, it is better to take even this old medication under supervision. Remember that the physician who treats himself has a fool for a patient.

How can we make ourselves cancer proof? We can't but there are a few basic dietary and lifestyle factors that can make it harder for the crab to snap at us. The general dietary prescription is that we should eat more fiber and starch, particularly the amylase-resistant starches. We should take a quarter of an aspirin a day; we should avoid too much saturated fat, salt, and alcohol. We should ensure that we get sufficient of the desaturated FAs found in fish, and evening primrose oil. We should avoid too much red meat, and margarine. We should reinforce our colonic bacteria occasionally with LAB by taking supplemented yogurts, or similar preparations. We should have legumes (not if suffering from a serious auto-immune disease), soy products, and fish several times a week if possible. We should also eat fresh fruit and vegetables daily. When we choose vegetables, we should favor the red, yellow, and cruciferous ones. Salad and cooking oil should be olive oil. We should avoid overindulgence in beer, cheese, and processed meats, but have the occasional (twice or three times per week) glass or two of red wine. And, of course, give up smoking!

Middle-aged women without gynecological symptoms should examine their breasts for lumps once a month, and have a pap smear every two years. Middle-aged men should have a prostate-gland examination once every five years. Both sexes should examine their skin periodically after a shower, and look for changes in appearance. That would make a good start!

Such a prescription would also help in the prevention of CHD. Cancer may have been the disease of the 20th century, but it is also during the 20th century that we learned most about it.

We have come a long way since Fibiger claimed that cockroaches caused stomach cancers in animals. His work was highly respected and he was awarded the Nobel Prize for Medicine in 1926. Today, in the 21st century, we know much more about how cancer is caused-more than any other generation, and so we have less need to be victimized by it. We know that it is a disease caused by an accumulation of genetic accidents. With careful management, we need not be accident-prone.

CHAPTER 6

THE TROUBLE WITH AGING BONES

Bone of my bone thou art, and from thy state
Mine never shall be parted, bliss or woe.
John Milton, *Paradise Lost.* 1667.

The thing about bones is that you are stuck with them. If you have a serious problem with your heart you can have a heart transplant. If you have intractable liver disease, perhaps you can get a new one, but there is not a lot that you can do about your bones. Sure, you can get a prosthetic joint like an artificial hip joint, but prostheses are an addition to, rather than a replacement for our bones, and as in some marriages, the union is often not a happy one.

We are wedded to our bones for life. Our skeleton begins to form on about the seventh week of our prenatal life, and bones are with us from that time on; sharing in everything we do for the rest of our lives. If our bones curve, we curve. If our bones give us chronic pain, we are in pain every time we move. Whether our problem is a dowager's hump, or chronic lower-back pain, bones affect our lives, for bliss or woe, in an intensely intimate and personal way. Our skeleton allows us to get around, protects our internal organs and central nervous system against damage, and acts as a mineral reservoir. Bone is an amazing material! It has to be strong or it could not protect, or withstand the mechanical forces to which it is exposed. At the same time though, it must also be light. It accomplishes these twin goals with an extraordinarily clever design.

Bone is actually composed of two quite different tissues. The first is cortical or compact bone, which comprises about 80 percent of the skeleton, and is very dense and strong tissue. It surrounds a different bone tissue trabecular, spongy, or cancellous bone. In normal, healthy bone, the cortical type forms the outer surface and imparts strength.

The insides of bones have, typically, a honeycomb appearance. The horizontal processes within the bone, which look like supporting struts, are just that. They are called trabeculae (Latin for small beam). They are reinforcing members and help to give the bone strength, without sacrificing lightness. Cortical bone is found mainly in the shafts of the long bones of the appendicular skeleton (shoulder girdle, arms, pelvic girdle and legs), but it is also in virtually every bone as the outer layer. Cancellous (trabecular or spongy) bone is found mainly in the axial skeleton (skull and vertebral column), and at the ends of the long bones. These trabeculae, in particular, can become very thin in osteoporotic bone, and can sometimes disappear altogether.

Osteoporosis is a pathological process associated with getting old, as is osteoarthritis, and these are the two age-related bone diseases that we will be considering.

Bones achieve enough strength to be able to cope with the enormous mechanical stresses which are placed on them, because they can rebuild themselves, or make themselves stronger when necessary remodeling. This idea, which we owe to the pioneering work of a scientist called Frost in the 1960s, means that bones can dynamically adapt to an ever-changing environment. External circumstances are always changing and therefore so are our bones.

The way that bones can be so adaptable is because hard bony tissue can be continually deposited or removed from the weight-bearing surface, as the need dictates. If certain bones are doing more work, they become larger and stronger-because the bone-making cells deposit more bone there.

If bone is not being used, say due to enforced bed-rest or paraplegia, then more bone is taken away than deposited and the bone becomes thinner. Bone remodeling can be positive or negative, resulting in a net skeletal gain or loss. Each year, between 10 to 30 percent of the adult skeleton is remodeled. It is necessary that bones be able to continually reinvent themselves.

They need to because they are working tissues and are constantly being damaged by micro-fractures. These have to be repaired and remodeling is the means of achieving this. There is however, another reason for bone remodeling. Bone remodeling helps with the maintenance of the body's mineral balance. Bones are a reservoir of minerals, called upon when needed.

Our living scaffolding contains two principal types of cells. There is the osteoblast, the bone builder (from the two Greek words, *osteon* meaning bone, and *blastos* meaning embryo or sprout). This constructive cell makes collagen, and orchestrates the deposition of calcium and phosphate resulting in new bone. The second type of bone cell is the osteoclast, the bone breaker (from *osteon* and *klastos* meaning broken). It reabsorbs bone by dismantling the collagen and dissolving the mineral crystals.

Calcium is an important mineral in our bodies, integral to cell signaling and many other vital processes. We need to ensure that our calcium levels are adequate. One way is through bone reabsorption. If, for example, someone is suffering from low blood calcium, a hormone is secreted by the parathyroid glands, small glands buried in borders and capsule (the outer portion) of the thyroid gland. This hormone stimulates the reaborption of bone by osteoclasts, which in turn increases the levels of blood (serum) calcium.

Bone reabsorption is also integral feature of bone growth where bone is removed (reabsorbed) from a non-growing surface and deposited on a growing surface simultaneously. At every stage in our lives, this most dynamic of tissues is always caught somewhere between the creation and destruction.

It is the balance between these two activities, bone deposition and bone reabsorption, which determines whether we are experiencing bone growth or bone loss. Up to the age of 30, more bone formation occurs than does bone reaborption. After around 35, there is a gradual loss of bone density as reaborption outstrips formation. Bone thinning, or osteoporosis, usually begins around 35 years. At first it is not much noticed, but as the osteoporotic process progressively continues, it gives some people bones so thin that they are highly subject to fracture.

Osteoporosis occurs both in trabecular and cortical bone. In the trabecular bone, the numbers of trabeculae normally decrease with increasing age, at first thinning, and then disappearing altogether. Bone loss from cortical or compact bone is mostly by means of the removal of bone tissue from the inner layers.

While all of us will not necessarily suffer from all of the age-related disorders which we will be discussing in this book, almost all of us, if we live long enough will suffer some degree of osteoporosis, or bone thinning, especially if we are women.

The rate of bone loss is different for cortical and trabecular bone. Cortical or compact bone loss starts at around age 40. Occurring at a rate of between half to one percent per year, it is linear for both men and women. Trabecular or cancellous bone loss starts earlier around age 35, and sometimes the mid-20s. It is also linear for men and women, occurring at a rate of 1 to 1.2 percent a year for men, and at a rate of 1.4 percent a year for women, but it is rapidly accelerated by menopause.

'Accelerated' certainly is the word to describe bone loss in women after menopause-a rate of up to 10 percent a year is common, 3-7 years after menopause. As a consequence, after 45 years, men in all age groups have more bone mineral than do women.

From birth till about 11 years old, girls and boys have the same bone mass. At the onset of puberty, girls exceed boys by 10 to 15 percent, with boys increasing during and after puberty. This corresponds to the general growth profiles between boys and girls, with girls showing a pre-pubertal growth spurt, and then tapering off, and boys growing more during and after puberty. The sex hormones are very important in causing an increase in bone mass.

Girls who exercise very vigorously during adolescence, to the extent that their periods stop, have a lower bone density than girls who continue to menstruate. In women, a slow bone loss seems to coincide with the decline in ovarian function before menopause, and this becomes a rapid bone loss 5 to 7 years after menopause. After that it tends to slow to the point where, by age 70, the bone loss of women and men is about the same. The loss of bone tissue tends to occur in women any time when an estrogen deficiency develops. Thus, if a woman has an early oophorectomy (surgical removal of the ovaries) or premature menopause, she will have a greater risk of developing osteoporosis.

Table 2: Overall decline in bone loss for men and women.

SKELETAL SITE	% OVERALL BONE LOSS	
	Men	Women
Vertebrae	14	22.47
Mid-radius	12	30
Femoral neck	22-39	~58
Second metacarpal	11	25
Ward's triangle	33	41

Osteoporosis is a more significant illness for women than men, as Table 2 shows. Moreover, women fare worse than men at all skeletal sites. In both sexes however, osteoporosis occurs at different rates at different sites, perhaps a difference in the proportion of cancellous to compact bone might have a bearing on this, but the main reason is probably that some bones are receiving more exercise than others.

We do know that bones that have a high activity level due to exercise experience less mineral loss. There is even a different rate of bone loss between different bones in the same individual, with those bones getting the greatest amount of exercise (weight-bearing) experiencing the least amount of loss.

Humans tend to have more bone on the right-hand side than on the left, while with rats it is the other way around. This is an inherited characteristic of all humans favoring the right hand side, irrespective of their hand of preference. Left-handed people also have more bone on the right-hand side. Most rats are left-handed (left-footed?) and they have more bone on their left-hand side.

Why osteoporosis occurs is not completely understood. We know that, it is related to estrogen deficiency, but aging men may also be at risk, as 30 percent of the hip replacements are given to them. Nevertheless, the incidence of osteoporosis in males is small compared to females, with an incidence ratio of 2:1 favoring the women. Healthy boys and men develop peak bone masses that are higher than those of their female counterparts.

Men start with more bone, and therefore can loose more, than can women, before the loss starts to become a disability. But notwithstanding this higher male bone mass, men also lose less bone than do women during aging. There is a link between the middle-age decline in female bone density and the abrupt cessation in the production of female sex hormones. Aging men also experience a decline in their production of sex hormone during their middle age, and men do get osteoporosis due to a deficiency of testosterone.

Just as women in menopause experience ovarian failure, their male contemporaries, experience testicular failure, however, for man it is much more gradual. One of the pioneers of osteoporosis, Fuller Albright pointed out, this winding down of male reproductive capacity, leads to an increased frequency of osteoporotic fractures. Male senile osteoporosis does happen, and for much the same reasons that it happens in women, but is much less common. In males, it can often be related to cigarette smoking, and alcohol consumption. Alcohol reduces the amount of circulating testosterone, both immediately, and over time.

Cigarette smoking is an osteoporotic risk factor for both sexes. Since heavy drinkers are often heavy smokers, and both habits contribute to the problem, perhaps in a synergistic way. Male 'osteoporotics', like their female counterparts, are found to benefit from sex-hormone-based therapy, in their case, the hormone that is used is, of course, testosterone.

Looking for mechanisms of osteoporosis is not a simple matter. As we have said, estrogen is a potent influencer of the condition. Bone cells have estrogen receptors, so it might be that estrogen acts directly on them by suppressing the osteoclasts and perhaps stimulating the osteoblasts, and, when this hormone is removed, the reverse occurs.

Without sunlight, or some other form of ultraviolet light, we cannot make vitamin D. This vitamin promotes the transport of calcium across the cells lining the small intestine and is essential for healthy bones. No sunlight, means no vitamin D (assuming that it is not available in the diet), and no vitamin D means poor calcium absorption, and therefore weak bones. A vitamin D deficiency in childhood produces rickets. Rickets was so common during the 17th century, that is was called "the children's disease of the English."

These English children did not get any sunlight, and their diet was poor. Bedouin Arab women, who are covered from head to toe, also often suffer from a similar deficiency resulting in soft bones. The richest source of vitamin D is cod-liver oil, a medicine despised by generations of children because of its revolting taste. Today, in industrialized countries, milk is fortified with vitamin D to the level of 400 iu per quart. The recommended daily intake of vitamin D is 400 iu, irrespective of age. In adults, vitamin D deficiency leads to ostoemalacia, or soft bones. This effects women more than men, and can cause the bones to bend or distort under the weight of the body.

According to one theory attempting to explain osteoporosis it might be related to the decline in production of a hormone. The hormone calcitriol, which is produced by the kidneys, decreases with age. Calcitriol is synthesized from a vitamin D precursor, in a reaction catalyzed by parathyroid hormone. By this theory, when the age-related fall-off in calcitriol takes place, there is too much parathyroid hormone (or hyperparathyroidism) because it is no longer needed in this conversion. The effect is to cause rapid absorption of calcium from the bones. Thus, it is proposed, aging results in an excess of the very hormone responsible for bone reabsorption.

Another theory is that estrogen deficiency may not act on the bones directly, but indirectly. An estrogen decrease prompts a decrease of another hormone, calcitonin (not calcitriol) that is produced by the thyroid gland. Discovered only about 30 to 40 years ago, it has weak effects on blood-calcium levels, where it operates in the reverse way to that of parathyroid hormone, tending to reduce blood calcium levels. So, according to this theory, a deficiency of estrogen causes a decrease in calcitonin, which then does not have its usual effect of causing calcium to be deposited on the bone. This theory is not a strong one, because the effect of calcitonin on blood calcium levels in the adult human is quite weak. The reason for this is that any reduction in blood-calcium levels from calcitonin, causes, within hours, a stimulation of the parathyroid hormone, which has the opposite effect.

Still other theories on osteoporosis involve the cytokines. Cytokines, we have met before, those inflammatory mediators? For example, interleukin-1, a cytokine, has a powerfully stimulating effect upon osteo-clasts (bone-munchers). Moreover, indomethacin, a drug used in inflammatory conditions, inhibits IL-1, and it also inhibits the bone reabsorption.

It is not known precisely why osteoporosis occurs, or why it is accel-erated by an age-related deficiency in sex hormones. One of the most promising lines of research involves cellular growth factors. It is thought that osteoporosis is not caused by an over-activity of the osteoclasts, but through a failure of the osteoblasts.

Cells are amazingly complex. They talk to each other by chemicals, which they produce. Different chemicals send different messages and one of these related to growth. When you have a wound, for example, tissue has to grow to repair the wound. Cells near the wound site tell the damaged tissue cells to grow, and they do so by means of chemical messages. After a time though, another signal must be sent out to tell them to stop growing, or the tissue would become cancerous. A fine balance is achieved by means of chemical messages. The chemical mes-sages related to cell growth are called protein growth factors.

Two of these are called insulin-like growth factor I and II (IGF-I and -II). A number of research groups have proposed that the changes in these local hormones might be responsible, at least in part, for an osteoblast defect, resulting in osteoporosis. Bone is one of the many tis-sues whose growth is stimulated by IGF-I and -II. They have a power-ful stimulatory effect on the osteoblasts causing them to increase in number. Defects in this system could certainly be responsible for an impairment of osteoblast function. But it is still not understood.

Minerals other than calcium might also be involved. One such is magnesium, which has a very important role in keeping our bodies healthy. It has a particular role to play in the prevention of mortality and morbidity from heart disease, where it helps to minimize the adverse effects of ischemia, and other types of injury. It is also impor-tant in maintaining the viability of our nerve cells, and plays a role in many biochemical mechanisms, including those of cell membrane flu-idity, and stability. One of the things magnesium does is to help avert the consequences of calcium toxicity.

There is evidence that magnesium might be an important factor in the changes that determine bone brittleness. Trabecular bone from osteoporotic women has been shown to have less magnesium than controls. Magnesium deficiency causes decreased osteoblastic activity and this would result in the cessation of bone growth, increased bone fragility, and larger bone crystal formation.

Furthermore, magnesium is essential for calcium metabolism. The two minerals seem to work together. High levels of calcium might not protect against osteoporosis without adequate magnesium. Estrogen therapy has also been found to increase the levels of magnesium in bone and soft tissue. One of the ways that estrogen might exert its important protective effect against osteoporosis is by making magnesium more available to the bones.

Certain diseases predispose people to osteoporosis. These include endocrine and metabolic diseases, such as diabetes mellitus Type 1, Cushing's syndrome, homocystinuria (an overproduction of homocysteine), hyperparathyroidism (an excess of the parathyroid hormone), hypovitaminosis D (a deficiency of vitamin D), and scurvy (a deficiency of vitamin C). As well as a number of blood disorders and cancers, such as leukemia, lymphoma, multiple myeloma, hemolytic anemias, sickle cell disease, and beta-thalassemia, as do some gastrointestinal conditions such as inflammatory bowel disease, gluten enteropathy, primary biliary cirrhosis, hepatic insufficiency, Wilson's disease, hemochromatosis, and malnutrition. Certain chronic inflammatory and renal diseases, such as rheumatoid arthritis, idiopathic hypercalciuria, renal failure, and renal tubular acidosis are also included.

As well, there are a number of drugs, which can also contribute to it, including aluminum-containing antacids, anticonvulsants, cisplatin, cyclosporine, glucocorticoids, heparin, methatrexate, plicamycin, thyroid hormone excess, diuretics (except thiazides), and alcohol. It can be also be exacerbated by certain other conditions including immobilization, osteogenesis imperfecta, disuse due to paralysis, Ehlers-Danlos syndrome, Marfan's syndrome, after organ transplantation, during pregnancy, and in Gaucher's disease.

If you have any of these conditions, or take any of those drugs, it is advisable to seek medical advice regarding the amelioration of their possible osteoporotic effects.

An individual's bone mass is, primarily, genetically controlled, but lifestyle factors such as dietary intake, smoking, and physical activity can contribute to variations in bone mineral content. The most important dietary-related risks for osteoporosis are a chronic deficiency in calcium, protein, and vitamin C.

Calcium deficiency at any time in an individual's life results in reduced bone mass, but how much calcium a person needs has not been settled. The recommended daily allowance (RDA) for calcium is 1200 mg for men and women up to the age of 25 years and 800 mg thereafter, but some argue, with a degree of justification, that the RDAs are too low (not only for calcium, but also for everything else).

The skeleton contains 25 g of elemental calcium at birth increasing to about 1 kg at skeletal maturity. The skeleton accounts for about 99 percent of the calcium in the body. The bones act as a reservoir for calcium needed and this element is constantly being removed and replaced. When this skeletal turnover results in a net loss osteoporosis and consequent fractures develop.

Women with hip fractures may have lost 50 percent of total body calcium. There have been many studies looking at the relationship between calcium intake and bone density in adults. The results have been assessed statistically establishing a connection between dietary calcium intake and bone density with a stronger relationship in premenopausal than in postmenopausal women.

Adequate calcium intake may have an even greater impact during development of peak bone mass that occurs in adolescence. It is therefore most important that adolescents and in particular adolescent girls have adequate calcium when the peak mass is attained at approximately 16 years. How much calcium these adolescent girls should be taking is not clear. One researcher, Lloyd, has suggested that calcium intakes greater than 935 mg a day will allow greater increases in bone mineral measures, but others believe that teenage girls should take supplemental calcium in the dosage of 1200 mg a day to produce a 6 percent increase in bone density, and thereby decreasing the risk of fractures, when they become post-menopausal women.

The National Institutes of Health Consensus Conference on Calcium in 1994 recommended that the daily calcium intake for elderly people be 1,500 mg, but also noted that adverse effects may occur with calcium intakes greater than 2,000 mg a day.

One of the problems with assessing the effect of dietary calcium on the development of osteoporosis is the paradoxical fact that those countries where calcium intake is the highest are the ones that also have the highest incidence of osteoporosis. This certainly suggests that while calcium intake might be important, other issues are involved as well.

Genetics is one. If osteoporosis runs in your family, you have a greater chance of suffering from it. Stress is another. Some research suggests that people under significant stress have lower serum calcium levels. And, s well, that people with psychopathology, or mental disorders, tend to have lower levels of calcium in their blood, and significantly more in their urine. This suggests that stress may make us excrete calcium. If so, the body has to compensate for this lost calcium, and the only place the body can go to make good the loss is from the bones.

Although how much calcium is being taken is important, so also, is whether or not you are excreting calcium. So what are the things, which effect our excretion of calcium? Sulfur-rich proteins (cysteine and methionine), salt and caffeine increase calcium excretion, while B vitamins decrease it. Fat, phytates (from fiber) and oxalates decrease calcium absorption, and sugars and calcium increase it. Many of these effects are small, for example, the caffeine in a cup of brewed coffee increases calcium excretion by about 3 mg, and this loss can be offset by adding milk.

Phytates are found in dietary fiber so the consumption of dietary fiber does increase our risk of osteoporosis, but the risk is only a weak one.

Cigarette smoking is a known risk factor for the development of osteoporosis. Women who smoke have almost double the risk of a hip fracture than those who do not. About 10 to 20 percent of hip fractures are attributed to cigarette smoking, which seems to lower estrogen levels. Smoking can interfere with estrogen metabolism to such a degree that some women who are on hormone replacement therapy (HRT) continue to lose bone, if they are smokers.

Heavy drinking is also associated with osteoporosis, as is cirrhosis of the liver, pancreatitis, cardiomyopathy, and brain damage.

Osteoporosis appears to be more common in Northern Europe and North America, than elsewhere, and different dietary habits and variable levels of physical activity and exposure to sunlight are implicated by this fact. One group studying the relatively low incidence of this disease in Greece suggests that a diet high in the monounsaturated FAs, such as those in olive oil, may be protective. Yet another possible good outcome from olive oil consumption!

This group explains the result by suggesting that the vitamin E content of olive oil might have a positive effect on the prostaglandins, which slow bone-reabsorption. Olive oil is so rich in vitamin E. that one group found that the waste water collected after washing down the presses, makes a very good antioxidant tonic.

All of us will lose some bone as we become aged, but some people will have an excessive amount of osteoporosis to the point where their bones will no longer function properly as mechanical levers. Furthermore, because osteoporotic bone is so thin, it fractures easily. The most common sites for fractures are the hip, vertebrae, and radius (forearm).

In most industrialized countries the cost of hospitalizing the aged, because of frequent fractures, is very high. Over 90 percent of femoral fractures, and 75 percent of all Colles' fractures (lower forearm) in the US are due to osteoporosis. Fractures of the femur (the hip), in particular, are associated with an enormous cost in the provision of medical services, as well as causing death and disability.

People often die soon after hip fractures, perhaps because it is such a profound disability, effecting in a fundamental way their ability to get around, or because of a combination of factors, including depression and the consequent lowering of the immune response, as well as postoperative infection. In the first year after a hip fracture, mortality is between 12 to 20 percent higher than in other persons of a similar age and gender. Many of those who do not die are unable to walk independently again.

Hip fractures are so prevalent because of the construction of the femur, the thighbone. This bone is the longest and strongest in the body. It supports most of the weight of the body, plus whatever we might be carrying. It fits into the hip (technically the bones of the pelvis are the hip, not the femur) by means of a rounded head, at the end of a narrow neck. In osteoporosis, the femoral neck, in particular, gets very thin, and since this narrow isthmus has the job of carrying most of the body weight, it easily fractures, usually after a fall.

After the age of 50 the incidence of hip fracture rises dramatically. Almost 50 percent of hip fractures occur among people 80 years of age and older, with women outnumbering men by 2 to 3-times.

In relation to osteoporotic fractures, industrialized countries spend the greatest amount of money on those of the hip, but Colles' fractures are more common among women in the United States.

However, it is neither the hip nor the forearm, which is most severely affected by osteoporosis, it is the spine. Most women over the age of 65 years will be lucky to avoid one or more vertebral fractures. Indeed, among the group of women at or over the age of 50 years, new vertebral fractures occur at nearly three times the rate of hip fractures, with 2 million white women being affected in this way in the US every year.

As a result of osteoporosis, the trabeculae of cancellous or trabecular bone become thinner and thinner, sometimes disappearing. When this occurs in the vertebrae, they at first become deformed, and then collapse, adopting a wedge-shape.

These vertebral deformities eventually cause the Dowager's hump posture; each complete vertebral compression fracture is responsible for about a 1 cm loss in height.

In Western populations, blacks generally have a higher bone density than whites, but among non-Negro populations the incidence of bone loss is not markedly different.

Osteoporosis is not a new disease. It has been found in excavated femurs that belonged to Nubians who lived in the Sudan in prehistoric times. The percentage of bone loss among the Nubians was similar to that of modern comparable populations, but the Nubian females had a much earlier onset of osteoporosis, between 20-41 years, than do modern populations. The group, who collected these data, has suggested that the observed early bone loss is probably due to nutritional factors, including long lactation periods (24 years over a lifetime), and more pregnancies than is usual in their modern counterparts. Both the lactation and the pregnancies would have lowered these women's supply of serum calcium, and the deficiency would have been made good by bone reabsorption, as calcium rich foods such as dairy products, were not as easy to find in the prehistoric deserts of Nubia.

Today, with modern nutritional practices the situation is completely different from what it was in ancient Nubia. The usual practice today of having only two or three births has been associated with increased bone density. Breast feeding in modern Western populations, has no effect on bone density, perhaps because the calcium supplementation is usually so rich. Menstrual cycle characteristics however, tend to have profound effects on bone density. An early start to periods, more years menstruating, and longer periods of bleeding during each menstrual cycle, have all been associated with higher levels of bone density of the distal radius.

Amenorrhea (an absence of menstrual bleeding), on the other hand, places a woman at risk of osteoporosis due to an estrogen deficiency.

Women, who exercise excessively and become amenorrheic, negate the benefits of mechanical loading on the bone from the exercise. If the exercise is reduced, and normal menses resume, bone loss slows.

Amenorrhea can also be caused by starvation, and, when this occurs in cases of anorexia nervosa it brings significant osteoporosis.

The major source of calcium in the Western diet is dairy products, but calcium is also in fruit and vegetables, meat, and other foods. Other good sources of calcium are cheese, sardines, and salmon (with the bones included). Vegetables do not have as much calcium as dairy sources. Of the vegetables, probably broccoli contains the highest amount. Other good sources are sesame seeds, almonds, rhubarb, oysters, and shrimp.

Too much alcohol is a risk factor for osteoporosis. This means no more than one drink per day for women, and two drinks per day for men. A drink represents 340 mL (14 ounces) of beer, 140 mL (6 ounces) of wine, or 15 to 30 mL (half to one ounce) of spirits.

Calcium supplementation should be discussed with a qualified health professional. It is relatively safe, but anyone with any pre-existing kidney disease should be very careful.

A high calcium intake in animals has been known to produce osteochondrosis, renal failure, and death. Reports of calcium toxicity resulting in death in humans are rare. They have been reported in milk-alkali syndrome (MAS), caused by a diet of milk and bicarbonate, which was popular among people suffering from peptic ulcers. Some of these patients took as much as 20 g of calcium a day. The symptoms of MAS include irritability, headache, soft tissue calcification, and renal failure.

These symptoms have also been shown to occur in patients with supplemental calcium as low as 1 to 2 g a day, in other exacerbating circumstances, such as use of thiazides diuretics, pre-existing renal complications, dehydration, and alkalosis.

Kidney stones are mainly made of calcium oxalate, and calcium phosphate. An excess of calcium in the urine (hypercalciuria) is a high-risk factor for kidney stones. Hypercalciuria is associated with high intakes of calcium and sodium, but low calcium intakes have also been associated with kidney stone formation. A diet high in calcium has also been shown to interfere with the absorption of other minerals, namely iron, zinc, magnesium, and phosphorus. As a result, a recent research group investigating the use of calcium as a supplement has recommended that calcium intake is kept below 2,000 mg a day.

The other important treatment for osteoporosis is estrogen therapy, or HRT (hormone replacement therapy). HRT is not completely risk-free, but usually the benefits outweigh the risks.

HRT is extensively used, not only to help prevent osteoporosis, but also stroke, and CHD in post-menopausal and oophorectomized women in the US and Australia, but is less commonly used in Europe and Asia. It gets a positive response from all parts of the skeleton, with both axial and appendicular fractures being prevented, at all stages of post-menopausal life, even in the very old.

Usually the estrogen is given with another hormone, progestin. Progestin, a synthetic form of the natural hormone progesterone, is added to estrogen in HRT for non-hysterectomized women, who would otherwise run an increased risk of endometrial cancer. It had been thought in the past that the progesterone part of the therapy had no effect on bone development, but views are changing, and it is now thought that it might, make a positive contribution to bone formation.

HRT carries with it increased risks of breast cancer, of fatal ovarian cancer, and of other cancers, as well as continuous bleeding.

The unopposed use of estrogen therapy (this would never be prescribed for a woman who had a womb) increases the risk of endometrial cancer, sometimes as much as 20 times. The risk depends on the dose and duration of therapy, but may continue even after the treatment has stopped. The inclusion of progestin has done much to neutralize this risk, as progestogens are known to reverse abnormal hyperplastic changes in these cells. There is a much greater risk of breast cancer from estrogen therapy than there is of endometrial cancer, however this association has been hard to prove.

One group of researchers has attempted to estimate the increased risk of breast cancer due to HRT treatment, and according to this study which included 100,000 women, the chances of getting breast cancer is almost twice as high than it would be if hormone therapy was not used. The risk of breast cancer from HRT has to be considered against the reduced risk of dying from other causes such as heart disease, stroke, and death after osteoporotic fracture. Mack and Ross sum up this risk by saying: "*Using the best available estimates, the contribution to mortality from estrogen-related breast cancer is unlikely to offset the protection against deaths from heart disease [136 p. 170-171].*"

I think that the jury has re-entered the jury box. What is the verdict? An increased risk of breast cancer is there, but the risk of dying is much higher if you do not take HRT than if you do.

HRT is not for everyone it is true. Some women experience unacceptable weight gain and other unpleasant side-effects, but for those who can tolerate the therapy, it should contribute both to the length and the quality of life.

A significant number of sufferers of osteoporosis do have malabsorption of calcium due to insufficient vitamin D. Some researchers feel that it is the principal factor leading to the disease. People with low levels of vitamin D have low levels of calcium absorption (from the gut), and compensate for this by "borrowing" calcium from the bones.

Many patients with osteoporosis have a malabsorption of calcium. Similarly, a significant number of osteoporotic patients show reduced serum levels of vitamin D, and it is very likely that this is responsible for the reduced calcium absorption in these patients, while some other patients have calcium malabsorption without reduced levels of vitamin D, and this could be due to a defect at the level of the gut.

Vitamin D therapy has been efficacious in the treatment of osteoporosis for some time. Chris Gallagher, an early authority on osteoporosis, said 10 years ago that: *"We have never seen a patient fail to increase calcium absorption after oral administration of synthetic 1, 25-dihydroxyvitamin D3 (vitamin D) [64 p. 395]."*

Many patients have improved on the combined therapy of vitamin D and estrogen, and tend to do better than those on estrogen alone. Therapy with this vitamin is perhaps the most common treatment for osteoporosis in the world. It has been used in countries, where the diet does not normally have high amounts of calcium, such as Japan, where more than one million women have been treated with great efficacy, and with few side effects.

The problem with this therapy in countries such as the US, Western Europe, and Australia, where calcium in the diet is not generally in short supply, is that after therapy, you can have an oversupply of calcium (calcium hyper-absorption), which can lead to too much calcium in the blood (hypercalcaemia). As we have seen, too much calcium can be dangerous.

Vitamin D therapy is useful in the treatment of soft bones, caused by a deficiency of this vitamin, but its usefulness as a treatment for osteoporosis, at least in Western industrialized countries, is not settled. Published reports over the past 20 years have found that vitamin D, and its relative calcitriol, can achieve encouraging results.

Early reports showed an increase in BMD by about 3 percent. A study by Tilyard has shown that low-dose calcitriol halved the fracture rate when compared to a group that received calcium but no calcitriol.

This finding supports an earlier study in the US, which also showed that calcitriol halved the vertebral fracture rate, and this was confirmed, by studies in Japan and Italy. In the US study, the fracture rate was reduced by 80 percent, when the patient was clearly a calcium malabsorber.

Very frail, very elderly people frequently have a vitamin D deficiency, because no one takes them out in the sun. These cases are typical calcium mal-absorbers. Most of the studies on vitamin D and osteoporosis have concentrated on such very old patients, who have had the disease for some time. For the rest of us, vitamin D treatment does seem to be a benefit in early menopause.

A French study found that it preserved the BMD up to five years after menopause, and a Japanese study produced a similar good result. In the Japanese study the women were oophorectomized, which is the surgical equivalent of menopause.

Vitamin D and its relatives stimulate the osteoblasts to produce new bone. As well, they enhance the intestinal absorption of calcium, and inhibit the osteoclastic action of parathyroid hormone. In addition to being useful in the prevention of post-menopausal bone loss, such therapy also helps with the type of bone loss caused by an over-secretion of corticosteroids (corticosteroid osteopenia).

Vitamin D has had good results in the maintenance of bone mass, and is gaining increasing recognition, inside Japan where interest in it is highest, and elsewhere.

Exercise is one of the best things we can do to decrease our chances of having significant bone loss. Bone is meant to work. Normally, it has to cope constantly with different patterns of loading.

A scientist called Wolff first suggested in 1892, that bone develops the structure best suited to resist the load placed on it. Mechanical loads make bone increase in size, and inactivity is conducive to bone loss. Since Wolff's time, many studies have confirmed his idea. If you don't use it, you'll lose it! Remember that!

One of the things we have learned about space flight, particularly over a long-term, is that it results in accelerated bone loss, as do other forms of weightlessness, such as professional divers might experience, and immobilization. The problem might limit the capacity of humans to travel very far in space, because without an exercise program they would be at severe risk of multiple fractures Exercising in a weightless condition can't be easy, but it is necessary.

Two researchers, Krolner and Toft, examined 34 patients required to take therapeutic bed rest for lower-back pain, and found that the bone-mineral content of their lumbar spine decreased by almost 1 percent per week. An even greater bone loss of cancellous bone was found among adolescent girls who had had to take bed rest after a scoliosis operation, and in patients with spinal injuries.

Physical inactivity results in bone loss, and exercise in bone gain. We know this from studying athletes. The X-rays of professional tennis players, examined by Jones and his group did, showed bones that were about one third larger on their playing side. Adolescent baseball players have better bone density in their dominant arm. It seems that what is important in using exercise to build-up your bones is that the exercise is a long-term one. The good effect of exercise on bone mineral content suggests that the sooner started the better.

Nursing home residents who exercised for 30 minutes a day, 3-times a week, experienced improvements in bone mineral content.

If you are severely osteoporotic, you will need to consult a physical therapist, or some similar trained professional, to determine the right type of exercise for you. For example, flexion exercises such as lying supine on the floor and lifting up your head should be avoided by people who have had spinal fractures, or are at risk of them, because of the extra vertical compression of your vertebra.

Reasonably healthy people should incorporate some exercise into a weekly routine. Exercise will build up your bone mass, and help you to avoid fractures by improving posture, strengthening muscles, and improving balance, and co-ordination.

Muscles should be stretched before use and a warm-up is recommended. Then when your muscles are nicely warmed, you can do some weight training. After weight training, the ideal situation is to finish off with a little more aerobic work. Weight training is ideal for building bone mass, but you have to involve as many bones as possible. Any good gym will have professionals available to help you devise an exercise program.

As we age our joints tend to wear and degenerate. If you can't ski for as long as you used to, it may be due to degeneration of the cartilage in the knee. Breakdown and degeneration of cartilage seems a universal condition of getting old. The worst form results in osteoarthritis (OA).

Several diseases broadly fit into the category; we collectively refer to as arthritis. These are OA, rheumatoid arthritis, septic or ineffective arthritis, and gout. Of these, it is OA that most people associate with old age, and it is OA that we will consider as a degenerative disease of bone aging.

Our bones are joined together by a mechanical system-called a joint, of which there are two types. The first is the synovial joint, where the bones come together in a cavity (containing synovial fluid, and therefore called a synovial cavity).

The word synovial comes from Theophrastus Bombastus von Hohenheim. Theophrastus, who deserved the second name Bombastus, as he often boasted that he was the greatest physiologist who ever lived, in his more sober moments, had the opinion, that what we today call synovial fluid, looked like egg-white. He therefore coined the name from syn- (actually sun a Greek word meaning with or alike) and -ovum, Latin for an egg. Thank you Theophrastus! You're a legend.

This fluid resembling egg-white has the function of both lubricant and nourishment to the cartilage (which itself has no blood vessels).

The synovial joint allows very free movement, and is the joint, which predominates in the limbs in places such as the knee and hip.

The other type of joint is a synarthroses. This is a union between bones without a joint cavity. In the synovial joint a protective layer of cartilage caps each of the articulating bones, and beyond this is the synovial fluid.

In middle age, everyone has some degree of joint degeneration, as well as the formation of small bony growths in the joint (ostoephytes). For some, these changes are quite severe, and cause considerable pain and restriction to movement. Such people have OA, the most common rheumatic disease, and one of the most common of all chronic diseases. It affects over 40 million Americans alone, and is not new. That sagacious Greek doctor Hippocrates knew of it and that it was an affliction of the aged.

Evidence of it has also been found in Egyptian mummies. It has been found in prehistoric remains of American Indians, and in the prehistoric populations of Mexico and Central America.

OA occurs where the normally smooth articular cartilage layer loses its elasticity and is more easily damaged by mechanical stress. The cartilage layer becomes pitted and frayed. Some cartilage repair mechanisms are then initiated, but eventually these too fail. The disease becomes progressively worse while the joint is being used.

Ultimately it becomes swollen, hot and very painful. The first signs of the disease are a roughening, and fibrilization of the articular cartilage. With time, this cartilage develops clefts and fissures. As the disease progresses, the articular cartilage erodes irregularly until it is eventually worn down. In some cases, the articular cartilage is completely lost, exposing the underlying bone. The bone becomes dense, hard and painful in such situations. While the articular cartilage is breaking down, there is an increase in the number of cells in the cartilage. Phagocytes, fibroblasts, and lymphocytes, invade the area, an inflammatory response ensues, and the joint becomes swollen, hot, and red. The injured cartilage swells, and is painful.

The bone cells respond to the wear and microfractures by growing more bone, and cartilage. So the bone tends to thicken at the ends, and new bone growths called osteophytes (also spurs, lipping, or exostoses) form in the joint. These bone growths often produce adhesions that make movement even more painful. In the joints of the fingers such bone thickening is known as Heberden's nodes. The name came for the English physician, William Heberden the Elder, who described them in 1802. Examination of autopsies has shown that this type of joint pathology can occur as early as a person's 20s. By the ninth decade almost everyone has some OA.

As anyone who has had this disease will attest, the main symptom of OA is pain. As well there is stiffness, and often swelling. The symptoms increase with use, and are relieved by rest. OA is not restricted to the weight-bearing joints. It often affects the joints of the fingers (interphalangeal). These are among the most common of the joints affected. Other common sites are the knees, the spine, hips, the sacroiliac, and the shoulders. Wrists and elbows are rarely involved. Almost everyone beyond the age of 50 years will have some evidence of this disease. Those who have it badly enough to justify a clinical diagnosis will be only about 5 to 10 percent. Such a diagnosis is rare before 40.

OA is more common and more severe with increasing age. In a lifelong study of the same subjects (a longitudinal study), the incidence of OA of the hand was 3.8 percent for subjects less than 40 years of age, 33.3 percent for the middle-aged, and 70.6 percent for elderly subjects. Age-related OA is particularly common in the hand, and its progression there is more rapid than in any other joint.

OA in other joints such as the hip and knee is less common, but is incapacitating there. As well, there is chronic back pain that can be caused by OA of the spine. In the United States the prevalence of severe or moderate OA is less than one percent for knees, with an additional 2.9 percent having mild OA there. The incidence of OA of the hip is 1.3 percent. The severity of the disease progresses more rapidly when in the knees than in the elbow, and more rapidly in the hips than in the shoulder.

The disease is initiated by an irritation to a joint. This irritation may be as a result of injury or due to excessive stress because of occupational habits, sports activities, obesity, poor posture, or simply the wear and tear of the joints in everyday life.

Several studies have shown that OA is more prevalent among craftspeople, farmers, heavy machinery operators, and laborers, than among salespeople, clerical and house workers.

The damage, irritation, or injury needed to initiate the disease might not be serious but is usually chronic. Stress to the joint resulting in microfractures is often overlooked. These are tiny fractures that occur after years of occupational or sporting bad habits. This is the reason why OA is so common among former footballers and foundry workers, people who put an enormous amount of stress on their joints. But you do not have to be a foundry worker to experience joint damage. It can happen to almost anyone, a jogger, or someone shoveling snow.

As with osteoporosis, there is also a close association between OA and menopause, an association recognized since the 1920s by Russell Cecil and Benjamin Archer.

Obesity is associated with osteoarthritis of the knees. Obesity tends to cause OA of both knees, rather than one. It is not sure whether or not obesity affects OA in other sites such as the hand and hip.

Heredity appears to have a role in the development of certain forms of OA, possibly through the inheritance of poor grades of cartilage. Several groups were able recently to demonstrate genetic linkage between the cartilage specific gene (type II collagen gene) and primary OA. This means that certain genes can predispose certain affected people towards this form of the disease through the inheritance of a particular type of articular cartilage. It has also been suggested that you can inherit anatomical abnormalities known to contribute to OA, such as congenital hip dislocation.

All human populations suffer joint degeneration, but certain groups suffer more than others. Of the different populations living in North America, The Inuit have the lowest incidence of the disease, and Native Americans the highest, with American whites and blacks somewhere in the middle. OA of the knee was more frequent in US blacks, while OA of the (distal interphalangeal joints of the) hands was more frequent in US whites.

Looking at other racial groups around the world, OA of the hands, feet, and hips, was less common among South African black females, than among white females, while South African black males had greater hand involvement than white males. It seems that Asian people do not suffer from OA of the hip nearly as often as occidental peoples and Indians. It might be that this disease least affects people who live in cold climates, such as in Alaska or Finland. It might also be that because the Inuit eat a diet high in fish that they are protected. We will discuss the importance of diet later. The disease however does not show a gradient due to latitude, as does melanoma.

These studies tend confirm that the people most at risk are those who do hard, manual labor. In a study of OA of the hand comparing two healthy Caucasian male samples, of urban professionals from Baltimore, and rural workers from the island of Brac in Croatia, while both had an increase in OA with increasing age the Brac sample had a significantly more joints affected, and affected more severely, than those in Baltimore.

Arthritis means literally inflammation of the joint, derived from the Greek word *arthron* meaning joint. The added suffix -itis usually refers to inflammation. The Greeks knew that arthritis was inflammation, however it has only recently been understood as such.

This sea change in thought about the disease occurred in 1975, when there came to Cambridge University two nonconformists, Ronald Jubb, a young Glaswegen graduate, and the grande dame of British medical science, Dame Honor Fell. They showed that cartilage was not as dead as shoe leather as had previously been thought, but was an active tissue. They also deduced that in OA the chondrocytes themselves, the cells that make the cartilage, were actively destroying their own handi-work.

Cartilage is a semi-rigid form of supporting tissue, made of proteo-glycans (a disaccharide joined to an amino acid) and collagen. Chondrocytes make this bio-cement but like an inefficient cement-lay-ers, they lay it all around themselves to the point where they get trapped in their work. Cartilage therefore consists of discrete chondrocyte cells, floating in a sea of proteoglycan/collagen matrix.

The modern conception of OA is encapsulated by the Bollet hypothesis that the underlying cause of OA is an injury to the chon-drocyte. This injury usually occurs in susceptible people by chronic stress to the joint. It causes the chondrocytes to make enzymes, and these enzymes are responsible for the break down of the cartilage. The theory is very well supported. Evidence has come from animal and human studies in which samples of the cartilage showed signs of the proteoglycan breakdown. In addition, some of the enzymes, such as cathepsin, have also been found in osteoarthritic erosions.

It might be that the collagen in the cartilage being subject to osteoarthritic attack is genetically different from the collagen in those who do not suffer greatly from OA. The degradative enzymes released by the chondrocyte attack do comparatively more damage to this (mechanically or chemically inferior) collagen.

Paradoxically the chondrocyte then makes a usually unsuccessful attempt to repair the damage that it has wrought. This happens because our cells cannot think, they merely respond to the instructions in the system software, the DNA.

The chondrocytes first turn nasty because they sense, incorrectly, that the joint has come under attack. They are responding to an invasion alert in much the same way as our immune cells do. However, after the cartilage is damaged, they then receive chemical messages that damage has been done to body tissue and must be repaired, and so, like the obedient little automons they are, they then set about trying to repair it. Usually however such damage is chronic and extensive, and beyond the recuperative powers of the chondrocytes, unless the initial injury is stopped and the joint concerned is given a period of rest.

OA is more common as we age probably because the structure of the cartilage changes. Twenty years ago, two researchers took cartilage from bodies in autopsy rooms and operating theatres, and subjected it to the type of testing used to examine the materials used in aircraft manufacture. They found that the cartilage from older individuals was significantly less strong than that taken from younger ones. The most likely explanation for this is that the collagen undergoes chemical change due to glyco-oxidative processes involving free radicals and AGEs. One such AGE is carboxymethylhydroxylysine or CML.

The peroxidation of lipids may be the main source of AGEs such as CML, and the main source of lipid peroxidation is ROS. The presence of AGEs in an oxidant and glucose-enriched environment brings about the reaction of glucose with amino acids in the proteins that make up collagen.

The accumulation of glycated proteins in collagen makes it hard and brittle. As well, it changes its color from white to brown, which is why this reaction is called 'the browning of collagen'. This change also affects the behavior of the cells on and near the glycated collagen. These begin to act strangely, in terms of growth, differentiation, motility, gene expression, and response to cytokines. These age-related oxidant products react with our collagen in other sites. This is why our skin gets loose and thin as we age.

The collagen in our joints does not escape this age-related change. You could say that part of the wear and tear which predisposes us to OA is the cross-linking of proteins in our articular collagen which is usually more common as we age and has the result of making our cartilage brittle.

As we age many of our weight-bearing joints change their contours. This remodeling, particularly in the hip and knee shifts the distribution of the loading, putting the maximum on a part of the joint which is not ideally suited for it, and it opens the site to capillary invasion, which brings to the site the inflammatory cells, such as macrophages, which can do further damage, particularly through the cytokines which they release. This increases the susceptibility to OA.

Let's now consider the sequence of events that take place in this disease. OA involves a joint under stress. It has suffered from microfractures caused by incorrect use. The chondrocytes start to wrongly read an invasion alarm, and they behave as though the joint had experienced a major injury or infection. The degradative enzymes are secreted by the chondrocytes that start to eat away at the cartilage. Capillaries start to be built to the site, so that the nutrients needed for repair can be brought there. Normally, of course, cartilage does not have blood vessels. As the site is injured, repair cells get switched on. Some of these are the cells that build bone, stimulated by the general call of injury being sounded in the area. The normal response of bone-building cells, osteoblasts, to injury is to lay down mineralization. So, the osteoblasts start to mineralize the joint cartilage. Synovial fluid and cartilage taken from OA patients has an elevation of pyrophosphate (a marker for mineralization activity). Cartilage does not normally contain bone, and to have it being laid down there is an abnormality, and a painful one. The joint becomes stiff.

Synovitis, or inflammation of the synovial membrane, then occurs. Because cartilage does not normally contain blood vessels, it is usually shielded from immune surveillance. It has what is called immunologic privilege. But, with the injury to the bone, the microfractures, followed by injury to the cartilage by the chondrocytes, this cartilage becomes a hive of cellular activity. Injured cells in the neighborhood send out an alarm call and this increases the blood supply to the area, as well as the number of immune system cells. Mast cells are activated and phagocytes enter.

This damaged cartilage loses its immunologic privilege. As well, some of the proteoglycans in the cartilage become antigenic or antibody raising, and the chondrocytes develop immunoglobulin on their surface. It is for this reason that if you take cartilage collagen from an affected animal and inject it into the joint of a healthy one you give the healthy one synovitis.

This takes us to the next stage in the development of the disease (pathogenesis), cell-mediated immunology (CMI). CMI is the typical inflammatory response to injury or infection First, the mast cells and monocytes move in, then the neutrophils, then the macrophages, and finally the lymphocytes. In OA, this cascade occurs as the articular cartilage breaks down. T-cells infiltrate chronically inflamed synovial membranes. Ultimately, what we end up with in osteoarthritis is a swollen, hot, red joint-an inflamed joint.

There is a lot of evidence to suggest that these are the events leading to OA. If you take fluid from the inflamed joint of a person with OA, you can find many of these cytokines and cells upon inspection. Furthermore, injecting into the joints of healthy animals some of the cytokines produced by an animal with the advanced disease has induced chronic synovitis. Cytokines produced by these immune cells have the capacity to degrade the articular cartilage.

Immunoglobulin (antibodies) and complement proteins are observed in degenerative articular collagenous tissues. The injured cartilage is itself helping to precipitate an inflammatory reaction in OA, which involves humoral (arising from the humors) and cellular immune responses. The immune cells attracted to the area, and the cytokines, which they produce, further degrade the already damaged cartilage. One of the concomitants of inflammation is the production of free radicals, which do further damage. This inflammatory response produces in the joint the cardinal signs of inflammation: the rubor (redness); the calor (heat); the tumor (swelling); the dolor (pain), and loss of function, symptoms that have become the signature of OA.

Elderly people (over the age of 40) can get OA in the fingers. The joint most likely to be effected is at the base of the thumb. Often it results in a bony, hard joint enlargement. The severe pain and inflammation in this joint can often be treated with the injection of corticosteroids directly into the joint. Almost all elderly people have OA in the neck, often severely, but only a small proportion have symptoms that require treatment. Treatment includes rest, which can be provided by using a soft collar. OA also affects the spine at the level of the chest (thoracic spine) and the lower back. Often this results in disc degeneration and the growth of spurs. OA of the hip, usually on one side, increases in incidence from the fifth decade onwards. This is often a painful condition, which makes moving an ordeal. For all these forms of OA, rest, immobilization, analgesics is the traditional treatment.

NSAIDs are used to treat a number of rheumatic and arthritic conditions, but can have some serious side effects including bleeding from the gut. So their use must be monitored carefully. There is now a new class of drugs that have just been developed called Cox-2. These can specifically interfere with the production of the bad prostaglandins (as do the NSAIDs) without interfering with the good ones (as do the NSAIDs). These provide relief from arthritis and rheumatism without the unwanted side effects.

Another thing that can be done is to cut down on your consumption of red meat products, and replace them with fish. Red meat products have high levels of Ar. A. This chemical gets converted into the 'bad' prostaglandins that tend to exacerbate the existing inflammatory condition.

Almost everyone over 40 has suffered from serious back pain from a number of possible causes. In elderly populations a common cause is scoliosis. Scoliosis is a lateral curvature of the spine. It is usually pain-less until degeneration of the spinal joints occurs at middle age. A common form of the disease is called idiopathic (of no known cause) scoliosis. This usually occurs in adolescents.

Primary scolioses are almost always linked to vertebral rotation in the growing skeleton. After the rotation occurs, the spine develops a compensatory curve in order to keep the head properly balanced above the pelvis. After the third decade of life, degenerative changes set in above and below the primary curvature. Scoliosis causes a limitation to movement. Certain movements can't be done without pain. Most sufferers learn to live with their disorder, adjusting their habits and activities accordingly.

One probably common though infrequently diagnosed cause of back pain is atherosclerosis. This condition leads to ischemia. In relation to the heart, this can lead to angina pectoris (serious chest pain), or a heart attack. When the abdominal aorta has significant atherosclerois, blood supply to the spine can be restricted. This may be particularly the case with smokers, because smoking also increases the ROS, which initiate atherosclerosis, while at the same time it reduces the levels of antioxidant defenses.

Perhaps another common cause of back pain is our minds. The back is susceptible to pain from emotional causes. Feelings of hostility, suspicion of others, anger, and resentment, can often be manifested in our backs by giving us a chronic ache. Are they feelings that we have turned our backs on? If so they have found a way to remind us that we still have some unfinished business to deal with.

Back pain is not a simple matter, many conditions can result in this symptom, so next time your doctor pauses to consider such an ailment in you, be a patient patient, he or she has a lot to think about.

What conclusions, if any, can we draw from all of the foregoing? Osteoporosis, we have seen is a degenerative disease that seems closely linked to the declining levels of sex hormones particularly estrogen and to lack of use. How do we prevent this age-related disorder? Obviously, start using our bones, preferably with weight-bearing exercises. Go ride a bicycle to thicken the neck of your femur!

Go to the gym, and do weights! Start to renew you acquaintance with physical activity. Keep in mind, that if you don't use it, you'll lose it. The severely osteoporotic, in whom normal exercise might do damage need physical therapy under the supervision of a trained therapist. Use alcohol in moderation and quit smoking. Make sure that your diet contains adequate amounts of calcium. Although calcium is most important during adolescence, it is still important later. People with low levels of calcium have more fractures, and lower bone-density measurements. You should be looking at a dose of about 1500 mg per day, but not more than 2000 mg. Avoid the calcium robbers-things that make you excrete calcium. Two of the most common are coffee and salt. Take adequate B vitamins.

Excessive amounts of dietary fat, fiber, and oxalates (found in tea) can interfere with your calcium absorption and so should be avoided. Magnesium is also important. After menopause, women must replace those lost sex hormones, and this may mean HRT.

Severely osteoporotic middle-aged men should discuss hormone replacement with their doctor as well. Finally, stop worrying! You'll never get out of it alive, anyway, and worry (stress) probably is a risk factor for the disease.

As well, you can do is to take fish oils, in particular EPA and DHA. These 'good' oils reduce the level of production of inflammatory mediators, such as the leukotriene. Not a lot of research has been done on this area of therapy but still some interesting facts have come to light. One group has found that the consumption of alpha-linolenic acid-rich perilla oil suppressed the progress of irritable bowel syndrome (IBS). Alpha-linolenic acid is a precursor to EPA, and IBS is an inflammation-mediated condition.

Another group has found that the high consumption of fish was linked with decreased risk of rheumatoid arthritis (RA). Similar good results may be obtained by the increased consumption of fish in the battle against rheumatism and OA, because OA, RA and rheumatism, all have inflammation as a principal cause. All this research is recent, but it seems that those cool oils from cold-water fish may extinguish the angry fires of inflammation. There is much to be learned about how N-3 essential FAs can dampen the inflammatory response. Given all that we now know, however, about the links between the consumption of fish to protection against CHD, cerebrovascular disease, and now rheumatic diseases, I am not be waiting for the research to come in. I am eating fish now! Bon appetit!

CHAPTER 7

THE AGING BRAIN

I can live with my arthritis,
My dentures fit me fine,
I can see with my bifocals,
but I sure do miss my mind.

Anonymous

People living in the world today have an expectation not experienced by any previous generation, and this is universal old age. Already the signs of global aging can be seen. This trend has been apparent in Western Europe, Russia, North America, Australia, and perhaps especially, Japan, for the past twenty years. This trend has been caused by a phenomenal improvement in early disease detection and medical care in most countries, along with improvements in nutrition, postnatal and neonatal care, social welfare and a declining birth rate.

This trend is increasing, as we, the boomers, enter very old age. Soon, most Western advanced countries will have to pay the huge cost of maintaining a very large population of very old people. If current trends prevail, between 15 and 35 percent of these can be expected to suffer from mental illness, and it can be expected that 5 to 6 percent might suffer from the form of brain aging, which results in the symptoms described as dementia. As medical and social advances preserve more and more people into extreme old age, the rate of dementia is bound to increase because some age-related changes in the brain seem to be universal.

Exactly, what will happen around 2030 when many of we boomers become ancient no one knows because nothing like it has ever happened.

Neurodegenerative disorders are increasing in the general population, and not *only* amongst the aged, and it is becoming obvious that they are caused by other, probably environmental factors, as well as by aging.

So, understanding the changes that occur in the aging brain is therefore a matter of urgency. In this chapter we will ask, is it possible to avoid the worst aspects of the neurodegenerative disorders?

The prospect of neurological deterioration is perhaps the thing, which we all most fear about aging. We all hate to think of ourselves as incontinent and confused, and reliant on others for the basic functions of life. This fear of aging is not new. Shakespeare who described it as second childishness said:

"Last scene of all, That ends this strange eventful history,
Is second childishness, and mere oblivion,
Sans teeth, sans eyes, sans taste, sans everything."

What happens to the brain as we age? It gets smaller. The spaces in our brains get larger and the stuff of which our brains are made, the neurons and glia, decrease in volume. According to Herbert Huang, it is not so much a loss of neurons, but their shrinkage, that causes this decline in volume. Aging neurons may suffer from a reduction in protein synthesis, and this may cause them to shrink, without necessarily being detrimental to either cell function, or cell survival.

So is it a case of *Honey, I shrunk my brain,* or do neurons die? As we age, some of the large neurons in the brain do shrink. There is a progressive loss of brain weight of about 2 to 3 g a year from the normal adult brain after the age of 60 years. Such weight reductions are probably due to shrinkage rather than loss.

However, there is undoubtedly some neuronal loss as well, and this occurs because of an age-related collapse in cellular respiration.

Although the degree of cell loss is not nearly as bad as was suggested by early researchers, there is no doubt that it does occur, and that in some demented people it can be quite substantial. Furthermore, this cell loss tends to occur in particular critical areas; areas of high activity, and especially in those areas of the brain connected with memory.

We can compare brain volume with the internal volume of the skull, which of course, never changes. Up to the age of 60 years, the ratio of brain volume to skull volume remains constant at 95 percent. It then starts to decline, being 80 percent for nonarians. In the time between a person's teenage and 60 years of age, the volume of the lateral and third ventricles (large spaces in the brain) increases from 15 mL to 55 mL. Indeed, some analyses have shown, a reduction in the volume of the cerebral hemispheres starting as early as 20 years of age. For men, this reduction is 3.5 percent a decade, and for women it is two percent a decade.

By the age of 80, the normal human brain may decrease in weight by some 15 percent, and much more for demented individuals.

The gyri (the ridges on the surface of the cerebral hemisphere) are thin, and the sulci (the troughs on the surface of the cerebral hemisphere) are prominent. There is a decrease in neuronal density, all of which indicates an age-related loss of neurons. In addition to neuron shrinkage and loss, there is also a loss of the tree-like connections between brain cells (dendritic arboration). This means that the tree-like structure of nerve processes (dendrites) often regresses, resulting in fewer dendrites from a particular nerve cell. Dendrites are extensive tree-like processes extending out from the neuron.

A loss of neurons does not necessarily imply a linear loss of function. We have learned from brain injury patients that our brains have a good deal of 'neuronal plasticity'. They can sustain a good deal of neuronal loss, without necessarily showing a commensurate reduction in function, because the brain is remarkably good at making up for losses, by intelligently employing the remaining neurons. Incidentally, we can make this *neuronal plasticity* work for us. Our brains are constantly changing, making new connections as we learn something. One exercise that can help to keep our cognitive processes intact is to keep our brains active. Try not to let a day pass without using your brain for something a little challenging. Your brain does not like to be idle.

Not all the cells in the brain are neurons. There is another type called the neuroglia or glial cells. They are not nerve cells, but rather the glue that holds the brain together. Indeed the name glia is Greek for glue.

One type of glial cell is the microglia. First described by Franz Nissl as *stabchenzellen,* or rod cells, in the late 19th century, and not properly explained until del Rio-Hortega did so in the fourth decade of the 20th century, it used to be thought that these cells are intrinsic to the brain, but it is now known that like most of our immune cells they originate in the bone marrow. These bone-marrow cells migrate to the brain during our embryonic development, and continue to migrate from bone marrow to brain throughout the life of an individual.

The microglia are *the resident immune cells* of the brain, but they were not confirmed in this role until as recently as the early 1980s. Like macrophages in the periphery, their job is to deal with infection, and clean up debris. A special glial cell, the astroglial cell, is star-shaped, and ensures that the environment around the neurons is benign. They remove any toxic or other chemicals that might harm the neurons. When a neuron is damaged, the astroglia increase in size and number to repair the damage. In the developing brain, the glial cells act as a type of scaffolding, or tram tracks, along which the migrating neurons travel. With aging, not only do the number of neurons decrease, but also do the number of neuroglia. In cortical areas, there is a decrease in the glial cell numbers of about 4 percent, between the ages of 20 and 90.

When you look at aging neurons stained by a particular method that makes them stand out, the Golgi method, you see a change not only in number but also some change in structure. At first the cell body develops an irregular swellings, or lumpiness, then, the dendritic processes are lost, and in addition the dendritic spines decrease. The latter are microscopic processes that appear on normal dendrites and help one neuron communicate with another. These changes mean that nervous transmission through an aging brain is less efficient as there are fewer opportunities for synapses.

One very important additional thing that happens to our brains as we age is that they get deposits of a protein called beta-amyloid. This protein is also deposited in other tissues, but its accumulation in the brain is a hallmark both normal brain aging, and of dementia; the only difference being the amount. The brains of people with dementia have more of it than do those of normally aged individuals.

Beta-amyloid often occurs in certain structures called neuritic plaques (NP), and neurofibrillary tangles (NFT). Once again, the more of these that you have, the greater are your chances of suffering a dementia. The key in all of this is beta-amyloid! We need to understand this protein in order to understand brain aging.

This protein, discovered by Scholtz in 1938, is derived from a precursor called amyloid precursor protein (APP), which is a vital ingredient for the construction and repair of membranes. One chromosome, chromosome 21, is responsible for the synthesis of APP. In each cell in our bodies, this chromosome is responsible for the APP needed for membrane repair.

Beta-amyloid gets deposited in blood vessels, forms in NP and NFT, under the linings of the brain, in sub-ependymal and subpial deposits, in the choroid plexus (pouch-like, blood vessel-filled projections of the inner layer of the brain linings, in the pia mater, and in the ventricles of the brain, which are responsible for the secretion of cerebrospinal fluid or (CSF). In the healthy aging brain, the appearance of beta-amyloid in arteries and capillaries usually occurs around the seventh decade, but it can occur earlier.

In 1981, a scientist examining brains at post-mortem found that there was an incidence of eight percent of this protein in the seventh decade, 23 percent in the ninth decade, and 58 percent after the ninth decade, although these subjects were from a geriatric hospital and may not truly represent the healthy aged.

High levels of amyloid deposits in the arteries of older brains seem to be associated with cerebral hemorrhage. Why the protein suddenly appears, usually in our seventies, has for a long time been a mystery, however later in this chapter we will explore a possible reason for it.

If you are lucky, all that you will experience is normal brain aging, which will lead to some, but not a highly discernible loss in your ability to think, and to remember. If you are not lucky, you may suffer a dementia.

The word *dementia* is Latin for madness, but that is not what it is. It is actually a progressive loss of memory and intellectual power due to a degenerative disease of the brain. About half of all the dementias are due to AD, and about one-tenth is due to small, repeated strokes. Dementias affect about 15 percent of the population over the age of 64 and 50 percent of the residents of nursing homes. Moreover, as the populations of aged people increase in Western countries, it can be expected that the incidence of dementia will also increase, both in relative and absolute terms, because as people enter very old age, their chances of acquiring dementia increases.

Autospy studies have shown that 50 percent or more of dementias may involve disease processes that are identical to that which we know occurs in the AD, but AD is not the only dementia. There are many other conditions that can cause dementia, including mixed Alzheimer's disease and vascular disease, multi-infarct dementia, PD, Huntington's chorea, Pick's disease, Down's syndrome, Creutzfeldt-Jacob disease, Parkinson-dementia complex of Guam, dementias due to certain infections such as syphilis, and others due to cerebral trauma.

According to US figures, and these would be similar in other Western countries, the incidence of AD symptoms is about 10 percent in people in their 60s, and 25 percent in people in their 80s. It may expected that 47 percent of those aged 85 and over will develop AD. AD currently affects four million people in the US alone, but within 50 years, this figure is expected to quadruple. AD is the third costliest disorder (after cancer and heart disease) with USD 82.7 billion being spent on it each year. It is expected that if the incidence of AD remains constant, that by the year 2040 this figure will have ballooned to USD 400 billion.

Patients with this disease start by having problems with their short-term memory. The little things of life, such as what television program was watched last night, or where the car was parked, begin to be forgotten. Afterwards they suffer more serious forms of mental confusion, and inability to think. Finally, they cease to think. The cognitive capacity of their brain is exhausted. Sufferers can continue in a vegetative state for about 10 years, requiring total nursing care before dying. The coma itself tends to bring on death from some other cause.

There may be a large pool of undiagnosed, pre-clinical cases in the community who have escaped diagnosis, either because they are still coping, in a manner, or are cared for by their families. AD does occur also in Down's syndrome patients, and indicative changes can be seen in the brains of some affected people as early as their 20s.

For AD, the pathological change is a large accumulation in the brain of beta-amyloid, usually in plaques and tangles, and much more than can usually be found in a "normally" aging brain. As well, there is significant cell loss, especially in the hippocampus, an area of the brain with importance for memory. The age-dependent cell loss during normal aging over a 50-year period is 27 percent while that in an AD sufferer is as much as 47 percent.

The disease gets its name from Alzheimer, the first person to describe such changes in the brain cells of dementia sufferers. In 1907, he described the formation of NFT, which, together with NP, are still regarded as hallmarks of the disease. Blocq and Marinesco originally described NP even earlier. NP, also called senile plaques, are dense cores of multiple proteins in sheet formation. Beta-amyloid is the main protein implicated in NP, but there are other culprit proteins, including tau, MAP2, and ubiquitin. Some beta-amyloid can also be found outside the cells, and is thought to be a by-product of the breakdown of affected cells.

NP are not restricted to demented brains, but can also be found in normally aging brains. In the normally aging brain, NP increase until the 9th decade, and then decrease, apparently reaching their maximum frequency between 70 to 75. There is a direct relationship between the density of NP and dementia. Most of the brain structures experience these abnomalities, but the CA1 sector of the hippocampus is particularly vulnerable.

NP and NFT seem to occur at about the same age in all populations, and across both sexes. These degenerative lesions tend to occur more in large neurons than in small ones. This means that they tend to occur in heavier brains than in lighter ones, since heavier brains usually contain larger neurons. Men usually have heavier brains than do women, but with the same overall number of neurons. However, the association between the development of these lesions and neuron size is not clear.

These abnormalities seem to apply up to the age of 65, before significant neuron shrinkage has set in. They reach their peak at around age 75-80, when shrinkage (also called atrophy from the Greek word atrophia meaning hunger) has begun, and then they decrease. Since these abnormalities particularly affect people with large neurons it may be that they appear only at the early stages of neuronal shrinkage.

It seems to me that there is one primary cause of the pathology seen in brain aging AD, and PD, and that is cerebral ischemia. Ischemia, as we know from the heart, means an absence, or a restriction, of blood supply. There are three ways that ischemia of the brain would normally occur. The first is by atherosclerosis in the arteries supplying the brain. The second would involve abnormalities of the small vessels and capillaries supplying the organ, and the third is failure at the cellular level. By this I mean, failure of the mitochondria. All three can occur in dementia, and to a lesser degree can be seen in normal brain aging, but it seems that the abnormalities at the level of the capillary and mitochondrion, are the greatest contributors to dementia, and are most advanced in patients with dementia.

William Osler, a Canadian Professor of Medicine, who in 1873 first identified platelets in the blood, in 1901, declared, *"man is only as old as his arteries."* This aphorism is as true for the arteries that supply the brain, as it is for those that supply the heart. Atherosclerotic thickenings in the arteries that supply the brain will, as with the heart, ultimately lead to a shortage of blood to this vital organ. People with symptoms of atherosclerosis in the arteries supplying the heart do not always have this condition in the cerebral arteries.

Some who have severe generalized atherosclerosis show none of this type of change in the cerebral arteries. As well, some people who have severe cerebral atherosclerosis have no symptoms at all, and no obvious lesions as a result. As we saw, the large number of immune cells such as T-lymphocytes found in advanced atherosclerotic lesions suggest that it is, to a large degree, a disease caused by our immune system, one related to inflammation. The same is true of cerebral atherosclerosis.

Cerebral atherosclerosis normally involves the main cerebral arteries, the middle, anterior and posterior cerebral arteries. A thrombosis (blood clot) that arises in the internal carotid artery will often occlude the middle cerebral artery. Such a situation can lead to ischemic strokes, and a type of dementia called multi-infarct dementia.

Another type of ischemia is caused by abnormalities in the capillaries. It is usually called micro-vessel disease. Cerebral blood flow is reduced in normal aging, but the cerebral capillaries in non-demented subjects are without significant kinking, tortuosities, or basement membrane thickening. By contrast, the blood vessels of AD patients have irregularities, including severe thickening and irregularity of the capillary basement membranes, as well as twisting, kinking and tortuosities of the capillaries themselves.

All fluids obey *the laws of fluid dynamics*. This means that blood tends to flow parallel to the sides of the blood vessel. This is called laminar flow, and all fluids driven in tubes with smooth parallel sides tend to flow this way. However, the blood does not flow with all the particles in cross-section moving at the same velocity. It flows with the highest fluid velocity at the middle of the vessel, while the lowest fluid velocity is at the walls. Near the vessel wall flow velocity is almost zero, resulting in a cell-free layer of serum. This is why nutrients trying to cross from the blood to the brain must locate themselves in this cell-free layer. Indeed, if they are to successfully make the crossing they must stay (or reside) there for a few seconds. This is called *the residence time.*

Any factor that interferes with this residence time impedes or prevents the passage of micronutrients to the brain. As we have seen, the capillaries of people with AD show abnormalities that include irregularities of the vessel lumen. This will result in turbulent rather than laminar flow in these vessels. Such turbulent flow results in shear forces on the lining of the vessel that can lead to injury. Also the cell-free layer is abolished where the turbulence is operating, reducing the resident time, and making it more difficult for micronutrients, such as glucose and O_2 to cross the to the brain.

Finally, going from the small to the very small, we find a third cause of cerebral ischemia-a failure of respiration at the sub-cellular level, what I describe as *Respiratory Collapse*. What is meant by this expression is that the mitochondria are so badly damaged by oxidant stress that they either fail to function at all, or do so inefficiently that they probably cause more harm than good. The main villains in this drama, as with other drama which we have discussed, are the ROS.

The human brain uses 20 percent of the body's O_2, and yet is only two percent of the body's weight. Although the brain has this big need for O_2, it does not have an especially good antioxidant enzyme capacity. Furthermore, the brain is largely made up of FAs. All that white matter is composed largely of myelin, and myelin made of membrane. So gram for gram, the brain would have more PUFAs than any other organ. PUFAs easily take up the unpaired electron that a free radical wants to hand to them. This makes the brain exceptionally susceptible to free-radical attack.

Certain parts of the brain are rich in iron, and, with a large amount of iron-rich tissue, neither the brain nor the fluid in which it is bathed, the CSF, have any iron-binding capacity. We saw earlier how under the influence of free radicals iron can leave the tissues in which it has been stored and become free ferrous ions, which in turn, powerfully stimulate oxidant stress. The neurons have a lower antioxidant capacity to the glial cells. Glial cells, the other cells packed around the neurons, do have some antioxidant capacity because they do contain some vitamin E. However, this vitamin E of the glial cell would be unable to protect this cell, or the neuron, in the case of a ferrous ion catalyzed, free-radical attack outside the cell, because all of the glial cell's vitamin E is located inside the cell in the mitochondria and endoplasmic reticula.

All the ways in which free radicals can produce damage in living cells apply to the neurons of the brain, only more so. Because the brain is such a big user of O_2, the problems associated with this use are magnified. In highly respiring tissues, such as heart muscle, liver, and brain, there are many mitochondria working furiously to produce the energy needed by the organism. The brain needs lots of energy because it is at work all the time. In order to supply this energy, mitochondria run their oxidative phosphorylation reactions constantly, but there is often a leakage of free radicals from this reaction. This leakage damages the mitochondrial DNA (mtDNA).

The mitochondria, those long-term boarders within our cells, have never surrendered their individual right to reproduction. In our cells, they reproduce themselves pretty much the same as they did in the primordial mud-pool. They have their own DNA and they reproduce by dividing within the cell. It is this mtDNA that gets damaged over time in highly respiring cells, such those in the brain. This often ultimately results in damaged and ineffective mitochondria, and when the brain's mitochondria are ineffective, the brain gets starved of energy. Like clapped-out old jalopies, the neuronal mitochondria bang away, but get nowhere, producing only smoke and noise, in the form of further damaging free radicals, in particular, and the superoxide radical.

Incidentally, the fact that mitochondria have their own DNA means that a mother who has experienced significant oxidant stress is likely to give birth to a baby that also will have faulty respiration. The reason for this is that all of the mitochondrial mtDNA that a child receives comes from its mother. So that if the maternal mtDNA is damaged by oxidant stress, the child will receive the same damaged mtDNA. This provides a powerful reason why young women of childbearing age should not smoke.

We do know that with aging there is an increase in the formation of superoxide ions. Aging modifies the conditions in the ETC, making it easier for electrons to escape without fulfilling the entire chain sequence. With aging our ETC becomes less efficient, especially in the brain.

How do we know this? In parts of the brain associated with high levels of synaptic activity, especially areas such the frontal and parieto-temporal cortex, cerebellum and hippocampus, there is, with age, a decrease in the amount of the last of the three respiratory enzyme complexes in the mitochondrial ETC. Under such circumstances, if the first two of the respiratory enzyme complexes are passing electrons down the chain, but there is less of the third complex to accept these electrons, then some of the electrons will escape the chain.

This leakage of electrons from the ETC is found in both aged and young animals, but aging, the leakage gets worse, and many more superoxide ions are generated.

When we discussed the electron transport chain within the Mitochondria we saw the oxygen the ultimate oxidizing agent was the final electron acceptor. This most reactive of elements is the ultimate destination of the electrons passed like hot potatoes down the chain. Usually, this reduction of oxygen results harmlessly in the production of water, but often, even in young people with good mitochondria, superoxide is produced instead. This process of dangerously producing superoxide, instead of water, occurs with greater frequency as we age, and results also in a greater production of the most dangerous of all free radicals, the hydroxyl radical (because superoxide reacts with water to produce it).

One of the few bodily defenses against superoxide is glutathione, and the level of this substance decreases in the aged brain. Further, we know that ROS produce damage to mitochondrial membranes, and further impair the ETC, so it stands to reason that ROS are likely to have their greatest damaging effects on the inner membrane where they are produced.

This inner membrane has some enzymes that contain copper and iron; metals that we know catalyze oxidant reactions. All of these events result in a reduction in the level of oxidative phosphorylation in aged animals (including of course humans). The respiration of synaptic mitochondria is detrimentally affected by aging, and we know that there is a decline in ATP production from pyruvate in the brains of aged monkeys. The loss of mitochondria through oxidative stress occurs in all respiring tissues, but the problem is worse for the brain, because its antioxidant activity is low compared with other tissues.

One of the natural antioxidant enzymes, mitochondrial SOD decreases markedly with aging in active parts of the brain. The other antioxidant enzyme, GPX, is also low in the aging brain, because the levels of reduced glutathione decline sharply in the aged animal.

This is because glutathione reductase, the enzyme that regenerates glutathione from its oxidized state, is also at a low level. The level of antioxidant defenses in the aging brain is still a matter of controversy, with markedly different findings on the levels of SOD, but most studies have found that older animals are less able to cope with oxidant stress, than are younger animals.

The mitochondria are not the only source of free radicals; one of the most common sources is inflammation. The brain, unlike most other tissues, is immunologically privileged. This means that it maintains a barrier to the marauding cells of the immune system, a barrier called the blood-brain barrier. This barrier is an obstruction to the passage of certain drugs and other substances from the blood to the brain cells, and the CSF. There are virtually no lymphatic vessels in the brain. The CSF, for the brain, does the function that the lymphatic system normally serves.

The blood-brain barrier prevents many drugs, toxins, and microorganisms, from reaching, and so damaging, the brain. However, as we saw with articular cartilage, immunological privilege is often more of an idea than a reality. Lymphocytes do find a way to reach the brain, and are able to cross an intact blood-brain barrier.

How can this be? A barrier only needs to be down in one small spot to be completely breached. The brain-blood barrier is not a perfect barrier; there are one or two small areas where it breaks down. One is the choroid plexus. Here the barrier is breached and inflammatory cells are able to cross over. Once these cells have entered the interstitium of the brain, local inflammatory processes take over, and the blood-brain barrier is then completely compromised.

Among the cells that enter the brain's tissue are mast cells. These secrete histamine, causing the capillaries to become leaky, inducing plasma fluid and proteins to enter the brain tissue bed (vasogenic edema). The release of enzymes by neutophils induces tissue damage. Inflammatory cells begin to enter the brain's interstitium by passing through the former capillary tight junctions, now made leaky by the histamine. Neutrophils enter this way. Lymphocytes just barge straight through the cytoplasm of the capillary cell. Monocytes and macrophages are capable of using either route.

In addition to these systemic immune cells, the brain has its own dedicated cells called microglia. These cells are small cells with finely branched processes, however at the first sign of danger to the brain, like The Incredible Hulk®, they metamorphose into huge lumbering amoeba-like phagocytes.

It is the abundance of free radicals, produced by the macrophages, microglia, and other immune cells, as their defensive weapons, that make inflammation dangerous. The most preferred weapon in this defensive arsenal is superoxide. These radicals rapidly get transformed to hydroxyl radicals, radicals capable of doing great damage to the susceptible membranes of the brain.

The brain, unlike most other tissues, is post-mitotic. The neurones lose their ability to regenerate soon after birth. The other thing that makes the brain different is that the substances that it needs for survival,

O_2 and glucose, can't be stored. The brain needs a constant supply of them, and is susceptible to injury, from a loss or shortage of these metabolites. Indeed, if any part of the brain is denied them for longer than seven minutes, it dies. When the brain experiences an inflammatory response, the neurons are often deprived of these metabolic nutrients because they are rapidly depleted by the unfolding inflammatory response.

Neuronal ischemic/hypoxic injury is almost always seen in inflammatory diseases of the brain. There are certain parts of the brain that are particularly susceptible to O_2 deprivation. These are the cortical layers III and V, the CA1 neurons of the hippocampus, and the Purkinje cell layer of the cerebellum. It is precisely these parts that are detrimentally affected in the aging brain, and to an even greater degree in the neurodegenerative dementias of old age.

There are some things we do know about the brains of people with AD that makes us comfortable in suggesting that ROS may have a primary role in the development of the disease. Firstly, we know that neurons with NFT (a marker for AD) have a high concentration of iron, and as we have seen many times, iron is a potent catalyst of oxidant reactions. Secondly, whenever you get iron, particularly in elderly people, you also get protein modifications in the presence of reducing sugars, and the production of AGEs. Thirdly, microglia, the brain's special macrophages, are activated and increased in number in the brains of patients with AD, and as we have also seen, where there are immune cells, especially phagocytes, there are free radicals. Finally, neurones with NFT show an increased concentration of aluminum, and aluminum stimulates iron catalyzed lipid peroxidation.

Evidence also exists that the brains of these people are experiencing respiratory collapse, as it was earlier defined. Glucose is the main fuel for the brain except in times of desperate starvation, when it may be able to process ketone bodies. If glucose metabolism can be shown to be low in the brains of these demented individuals, then so is respiration, because respiration in the brain is nothing other than the oxidation of glucose.

Indeed, this can be shown, by means of a high-tech imaging device, called Positron Emission Topography, or PET. When this instrument is used to look at the brains of people with dementia, or those developing it, what you see is a significant decline in the amount of glucose being metabolized in the frontal cortex, the parietal cortex, and the hippocampus. The evidence for this is overwhelming. Indeed, at an early stage of AD, one of the areas to suffer most from poor glucose metabolism is the prefrontal cortex, which is crucial for memory, as is the hippocampus.

One European research group, Meier-Rugge and colleagues, recently showed that when you compare the amount of glucose being metabolized in demented brains to that being metabolized in healthy brains of the same age, there is a 70 percent decline in glucose turnover. The brains of people with dementia have only about 30 percent the amount of glucose metabolism that can be seen in the brains of the healthy aged.

The brain can live with the reduction of glycolysis that occurs in normal aging, that is to say, to about 40 percent of peak rates, but it can't live successfully with the subsequent reduction that occurs in dementia. This group have called a glycolysis level of 40 percent of peak rates as the brain's functional reserve capacity. Accordingly, when this reserve capacity is exhausted, the individual concerned must show the symptoms of dementia.

Why is there a substantial drop in levels of glycolysis in aged and demented brains? Glucose is oxidized to produce energy, and that the greatest amount of energy from the oxidation of glucose is in the aerobic phase, when pyruvate is fed to the mitochondria. If people with dementia have low levels of glucose metabolism, that suggests that their mitochondria are no longer functional, in other words, that they have experienced respiratory collapse. The brain mitochondria are so damaged by ROS that they are hardly able to function.

How then does the production of beta-amyloid fit into this picture? Beta-amyloid precursor protein (APP) is normally synthesized by chromosome 21. Without APP we could never have the repair and regeneration of our cell membranes in the liver, kidney, muscles or brain. APP is a vital protein for membrane repair and regeneration everywhere. Meier-Rugge and colleagues have pointed out that APP is normally integrated into the cellular membranes. When it is needed for repair, it is split from the membrane by enzymes called proteases.

If cellular energy (ATP) is low, due to a decreased glucose turnover, this reaction does not go ahead. APP cannot be split from the membrane, and cannot be used to repair cell membranes. If APP is not used for cellular repair, beta-amyloid starts to build-up in the neuronal membranes, resulting in its incorporation into NP and NFT.

So if you will, the build-up of beta-amyloid is a symptom or a signal that the brain's respiration is faulty. That is why this protein can be found in the normally aged brain, because all of us have a decrease in respiratory function as we age, it is part of the wear and tear of aging. However, in demented patients, there is a widespread breakdown of cellular respiration, and therefore proportionately more beta-amyloid."In short, the accumulation of beta-amyloid is a sign that the brain is running out of energy.

What would have happened if the cell had sufficient energy? In such a case, the beta-amyloid precursor protein would have been split-off and used. There would be no beta-amyloid left in the membrane. When this does not happen, an intact beta-amyloid molecule remains in the membrane. These accumulate in senile plaques, and in the vessel walls.

Once the deposition of beta-amyloid starts to occur, the process can then be self-sustaining.. Beta-amyloid is a neurotoxin, and its toxic qualities arise because it increases the production of

H_2O_2 , and so, the production of lipoperoxides. We can prove this by adding antioxidants, such as vitamin E, to cultures containing beta-amyloid.

When this is done, the antioxidant reduces both the H_2O_2 levels, and the neurotoxicity of beta-amyloid. This is why people with a large accumulation of beta-amyloid get progressively worse. At first, the beta-amyloid forms, as we have said, due to respiratory collapse. There is insufficient cellular energy to use it up. Once it begins to accumulate however, a secondary process ensues, namely it generates even more damaging ROS, which in turn cause further respiratory collapse of the mitochondria, and so the situation gets progressively worse. This results in the patient having greater and greater cognitive difficulty, because of greater and greater brain damage.

In addition to this, the deposition of beta-amyloid may also be related to immune system dysfunction. It has been known since the 1960s that when researchers killed off cells of the thymus gland in experimental animals, that they also enhanced the production of beta-amyloid. Furthermore, if the T-cells in these animals were stimulated, there was less beta-amyloid production. We know that in aging our functional thymus tissue decline markedly, mainly due to the deleterious effects of stress hormones. When this happens, beta-amyloid forms more easily.

It is common that people with dementia-related disorders, do not have a global disorder, but have a disorder that targets particular neurones, especially ones that use the neurotransmitter acetylcholine (ACh). This has been known since 1964, when Pope and his colleagues, first reported that acetylcholinesterase, the enzyme that breaks down ACh after it has been used in neural transmission, was lower in people with AD.

In 1980, this observation was extended to other dementias, including adult patients with Down's syndrome, alcoholic dementia, and Cruetzfeldt-Jakob disease. It has been found that the cognitive problems seen in these patients might be in large part ascribed to a loss of neurones using this neurotransmitter in the neocortex and hippocampus.

The reason why these dementias seem mostly to effect neurones using one particular neurotransmitter can also be traced to failure of respiration-or a failure in how the brain gets its energy from glycolysis. ACh is made from a chemical called acetylcoenzyme A. This is the key substrate for the synthesis of ACh. In the brain, acetylcoenzyme A is synthesized from glycolysis only. If glycolysis is down regulated, because of respiratory collapse, then there would be much less acetylcoenzyme A available for the synthesis of ACh. So it is that the cholinergic neurons suffer the most from respiratory collapse, since the reduction in glucose metabolism means that they are no longer supplied with their neurotransmitter.

How does oxidant damage cause respiratory collapse? When membranes are oxidized, they become hard or stiff. A stiff or hard membrane upsets the capacity that cells normally have of talking to each other (signal transduction). The first sign that the cell has that it is in distress is that its signal transduction no longer operates, as it should. For signal transduction to operate correctly, the membrane needs to be fluid. In normal aging, as a result of the oxidant stress to which we are all subject, there is a loss of membrane fluidity, and therefore some loss of cell signaling capability. This process would be happening in all the aging membranes, the plasma membrane as well as the membranes in and around organelles, such as those in and around the mitochondrion. The mitochondrion could be expected to suffer from most from oxidant stress, firstly because it handles molecular O_2 and has a highly active ETC, secondly because it is made up almost entirely of membranes.

Membranes under this sort of oxidant attack try to remedy the situation, but this only makes matters worse. They try to raise their fluidity by using the enzyme phospholipase A_2. Phospholipase A_2 is normally used by the cell to split arachidonic acid from the cell membrane, the first step in prostaglandin synthesis.

The mammalian membrane is composed of three major classes of lipids: phospholipids, glycolipids, and cholesterol. Phospholipids, the main constituent of membranes, are elongated tad-pole shaped molecules with a water soluble polar group at one end, the head end, and a water hating or hydrophobic tail composed of fatty acids.

Remember that we talked about membranes as being amphiphatic, which means soluble in both water and oil. This is the reason why membranes have this characteristic. It accounts for the observation of Ben Franklin in 1773 that *"When you put (a drop of oil) on water, it spreads instantly, many feet around, becoming so thin as to produce the prismatic colors, for a considerable space..."*

The hydrophobic tail end of the phospholipid is composed mainly of fatty acids. The type of FAs that form the FA tail of the phospholipids determines the softness or fluidity in the membranes of most animal cells. If there is a predominance of saturated fatty acids, the membrane is rigid, whereas UFAs in a high proportion, favor a softer or more fluid membrane. In humans and other mammals however, the key regulator of membrane fluidity is cholesterol.

Even in mammals, however, you can make membranes harder by feeding the subject with SaFAs. This causes their incorporation into the membrane phospholipid. Experiments involving the feeding of SaFAs to mice have revealed that when the incorporation of saturated fatty acids reduces the membrane UFAs to 50 percent or less, that the cell growth is severely inhibited. This is because such a large amount of SaFAs in the cell membrane reduces membrane fluidity to the point where continued growth becomes impossible.

A similar effect is obtained if you oxidize the membrane lipids. Lipid peroxidation makes membranes harder, because it oxidizes the membrane FAs. This induces rigidity in the membrane because the lipid molecules can't rotate; an effect called steric hindrance.

These oxidant changes affect synaptic membranes and mitochondria more than they do relatively quiescent membranes, and the use of phospholipase A_2 by cell and mitochondrial membrane is a desperate last resort to make the membrane softer.

With mitochondria in particular, we know that superoxide leaked from the inner membrane stimulates phospholipase A_2 action. However, all membranes under oxidant stress release phospolipase A_2. This causes the membrane to begin to fill with UFAs, such as LA and DHA. In an oxidant environment, this strategy by the cell only makes the situation worse. The high preponderance of UFAs in a membrane in an oxidant environment provides yet more substrate for the lipid peroxidation reactions. Thus, the membrane's desperate attempt to remedy its perilous situation only results in further lipid peroxidation. The lipid peroxides so formed may be the main destructive elements in mitochondrial damage seen under conditions of oxidant stress.

We know from laboratory experiments that a variety of pro-oxidants cause Ca^{2+} to be released by mitochondria. Mitochondria normally have an extremely high capacity for safe storage Ca^{2+} in the cell, but when they have been damaged by oxidant stress this does not happen. These two events, the stimulation in the mitochondrial membrane of phospholipase A_2, and the release of Ca^{2+} by the mitochondrion, puts the mitochondrion on a downward a spiral to death. Ca^{2+} ions become excessively cycled (continuously taken up and released) by the damaged mitochondria causing the inner membrane to become damaged. That inner membrane is where the oxidative phosphorylation reactions take place, the precious cascade of events that provides energy for the cell to function. The Ca^{2+} cycling leads to a decreased ability of mitochondria to retain Ca^{2+}, by an uncoupling of mitochondria from their oxidative phosphorylation activity, and an impairment, if not a total breakdown of ATP synthesis. When this happens to many of the mitochondria, it is not only the mitochondria, but also the cell itself that is in dire straits.

The only things that could have saved the cell would have been the Ca^{2+}/ATPase pumps, cellular pumps located in the membrane, which like ballast pumps on a ship have the job of pumping excess out, but these depend on ATP to work, and if the mitochondria are not properly producing ATP, they are out of commission. So, when this type of damage is widespread, there is nothing to prevent the inward rush of gloom, and the ship goes down. The ensuing rise of Ca^{2+} ions within the cell cannot be counterbalanced by buffering from the damaged mitochondria, which under normal circumstances, would act as a safety device preventing any extreme increase in the cytoplasmic Ca^{2+} concentration.

The cell goes into a deadly paroxysm; Ca^{2+}-cycling and ATP depletion together become the joint trigger for apoptosis, or cellular suicide. The final cellular dance of death, apoptosis, involves dissipation of GSH, and, the loss of electrical properties within the inner mitochondrial membrane. In its final desperatemilliseconds of life, the cell produces a final, frenetic and deadly production of free radicals, then totally loses its ability to maintain it healthy low Ca^{2+} levels. This element then swamps its vital processes that stop functioning entirely. That cell is no more!

Looking at the process, it is clear that although the mitochondrial membranes are directly injured by a synergistic interaction between calcium influx and ROS, it is the production of the enzyme phospholipase A2 that is the key to this final expiration.

We know this, because if you inhibit this enzyme, even in the presence of Ca^{2+} and ROS, you can protect mitochondrial membranes from damage.

The role of oxidant stress in mitochondrial collapse, and therefore ultimately cellular collapse, is borne out by certain experiments involving natural toxins. A bacterial alkaloid, called staurosporine, when used to treat cells in culture, has been found to make them commit suicide (programmed cell death or apoptosis). It seems that staurosporine-induced apoptosis engages a cell in a deadly process involving ROS production, oxidant stress and mitochondrial dysfunction. However, when vitamin A, an antioxidant is added, the degree to which this apoptosis occurs is significantly reversed. Moreover, the production of mitochondrial ROS was increased 4.4 times in culture by the staurosporine-treatment, and reduced to only a twofold increase when the vitamin was added, so it is reasonable to assume that staurosporine causes apoptosis by means of stimulating ROS production. A similar reversal of this process has been produced by other natural antioxidant enzyme systems, such as SOD. This raises an intriguing possibility. Staurosporine might provide a model for what happens to the brain during aging and dementia. Staurosporine stimulates the production of ROS and the consequent high state of oxidant stress then leads to apoptosis or cellular death.

We know that in an aging brain there is no shortage of ROS, so it is very likely that this natural circumstance also leads to apoptosis, in the same way. But will antioxidant treatment prevent the damage to the brain occurring with aging, as it does with staurosporine treatment? If it does, then we might have a treatment for brain aging, and possibly dementia as well. The answer to this question will have to wait until all the appropriate clinical trails have been done, and that could take many years. In order to be conclusive, such trials would have to be longitudinal, that is, conducted over at least 20 years. My advice is: don't wait for the trials, take your antioxidants now!

The importance of immune responses in the disease processes of aging cannot be overstated. Inflammation has been associated with AD for some time. We know that: a connection exists between rheumatoid arthritis and AD; there is some response in AD patients to the use of anti-inflammatory agents; the presence of activated micoglia have been found in CNS tissue for all of these dementia related disorders. They have also been found in tissues from PD patients, and in another dementia disease, amyotrophic lateral sclerosis (ALS). Inflammatory immune cells have been found near the dying neurons and lesions of people with AD. So the evidence connecting inflammation and dementia diseases is strong.

Not only is it known that in some way inflammation contributes to age-related dementia diseases, but perhaps it is a special type of inflammation that is involved, the auto-immune response, where immune cells (B-lymphocytes) raise antibodies against our own cells, or substances connected with them. An autoimmune response is found in patients with AD, but not in Down's syndrome patients.

The reason for this is probably that the AD patients are generally older, and autoimmune antibodies rise with aging, especially anti-brain antibodies. Many different types of autoantibodies have been found in the CSF and sera of these patients. These include anti-brain antibodies, anti-cholinergic antibodies, anti-pituitary cells antibodies, anti-neurone-axon filament proteins, anti-myelin basic protein, anti-microglial antibodies, anti-astocyte antibodies, and anti-beta-amyloid protein antibodies. These must have a potent effect, yet to be determined.

It is my view that oxidant stress and autoimmunity work together. It might be for example, that beta-amyloid is formed in various lesions as a result of respiratory collapse, as we have described, and then, because it is toxic, and antigenic, B-lymphocytes raise antibodies against it. The immune system of elderly people is more likely to do this because with aging clonal deletion fails, and the body is increasingly unable to distinguish self from non-self. Indeed, even the age-related regression of the thymus gland, responsible for the failure of clonal deletion, is itself an example of apoptosis, and probably caused by a similar oxidant stress induced mechanism. The autoantibodies so formed attack the brain cells, and finish them off.

Oxidant stress is also implicated as a possible cause for PD. PD is a neurodegenerative disorder characterized by progressive cell loss, mostly to dopaminergic neurones of the substantia nigra. Several factors, including oxidant stress and decreased activity of complex I of the mitochondrial respiratory chain, are involved in the degenerative process. Let's look at the possible mechanism for this collapse.

In PD, dopaminergic cell death in the substantia nigra is associated with a profound deficiency of GSH. This results in mitochondrial dysfunction. The fall in GSH seems to occur before the mitochondrial dysfunction and cell death, and might be the cause. Merad-Boudia and colleagues found a crucial role for GSH in maintaining the integrity of mitochondrial function in neuronal cells. These researchers have found oxidant stress can lead to mitochondrial impairment that in turn leads to a fragmentation of the mtDNA. But the whole cascade of events seems to be initiated by GSH depletion.

Is there any evidence for a hypothesis that places oxidant stress at center stage in our thinking about PD? Apart from the low levels of GSH, which in itself suggests oxidant stress, there are other factors.

Measurements from the substantia nigra of patients with advanced PD, just before these cells died, have shown that these cells also demonstrate an increase in: lipid peroxidation; superoxide dismutase activity; and/or free iron levels. All of these betray the smoking gun of oxidant stress involvement in the development of PD.

It seems that low levels of GSH make brain cells, and in particular those of the substantia nigra, susceptible to destruction by toxins, the endogenous ones that we make ourselves and exogenous ones, which we introduce to ourselves. GSH is a potent free-radical scavenger in the brain, and its decrease in the brains of PD patients has been interpreted as a higher degree of oxidant stress in these people.

The dopaminergic neurones, in places like the substantia nigra, are particularly susceptible to damage by H_2O_2. The production of dopamine from these neurones requires ATP. If the mitochondria in this area have had a respiratory collapse, they would then be unable to supply the ATP for the dopamine release. H_2O_2 seems to be so important in this disease because it is known to inhibit the ATP synthesase complex, the enzyme involved in ATP production. It seems that as the brain experiences oxidant stress induced by the exposure to H_2O_2, there is an inhibition of the uptake of dopamine by the presynaptic neurones. What might happen then, is that the dopamine would break down, giving rise to further oxidant stress, ultimately causing the death of the striatal and nigral cells, through some of the events, which we have described earlier. H_2O_2 is probably the initiator, but a gradual dissolution of the dopamine producing neurons then takes place, due to a combination of factors, not the least of which is *respiratory collapse* of the neuronal mitochondria.

What of alcohol? Why is it that alcoholics often seem to suffer from dementia? We know from studies with animals that those animals, which have been chronically fed alcohol, have developed a deficiency of GSH in the mitochondria as well, just like the PD patients. Alcohol has this effect when taken in excess because it can interfere with a particular carrier responsible for taking glutathione from the cell, and transferring it into the mitochondrial matrix.

The GSH depletion so developed, then causes the cell so affected to be more seriously damaged by oxidant cytokines, such as tumor necrosis factor. The nature of this specific carrier has not yet been discovered.

There are other hypotheses related to the causes of the neurodegenerative disorders of aging. One attributes the generation of beta-amyloid to neurological toxins, ingested or produced internally. It does not, however, explain why it is that certain parts of the brain seem to avoid the deposition of beta-amyloid entirely. If beta-amyloid is the result of a globally acting toxin, it should be deposited in similar quantities everywhere.

Using the Meier-Rugge hypothesis, we can explain why some parts of the brain seem more affected than others, because they are more dependent on respiratory processes than are others; they are more metabolically active. Examples of this are the synaptic parts of the neurones. These have a high level of metabolic activity, and also have a high level of beta-amyloid deposition. The highest level of oxidant stress is associated with areas that are high in trace metals. Certain parts of the brain are higher iron and copper than others.

Aluminum is another metal that has often been found to be raised in the brains of people with AD. Humans consume about 30 mg a day of this metal, on average, through water, food, and drugs. There is, in addition to this intake, some contribution made by the use of aluminum cooking appliances, especially in Asia where such utensils are popular. There is also some contribution made to our aluminum load from the use of aluminum foils for food wrapping and preparation. Aluminum can do damage, both by stimulating the iron catalyzed oxidant reaction, and because it is itself a well-known neurotoxin.

It is thought that people with AD have a genetic susceptibility towards altered function of a protein called transferrin. This is a protein used to eliminate aluminum. Because of that, this metal tends to accumulate in those people, and because it is cytotoxic, this ultimately results in neuronal death.

Zinc is another metal, which in high concentrations can result in beta-amyloid deposition. Certain parts of the brain, such as the synaptic terminals and the hippocampus, have a relatively high zinc concentration, and these are also areas where there is a high degree of beta-amyloid deposition in AD. It seems that those people who tend to suffer from dementia have abnormal zinc metabolism. This abnormality results in high extracellular levels, and low intracellular levels of zinc in their brains.

It is known that patients with AD often have serum homocysteine levels higher than those in aged-matched controls. An increase in serum homocyteine has been identified as an early marker of the disease. Not only that, but they also have low levels of vitamin B_{12} and folate. What is happening, it seems, is that such dementia-prone patients have an abnormal amino acid metabolism. They are unable to effectively metabolize homocysteine, and it accumulates. In doing so, it is adding to their problems, because it is toxic and highly atherosclerotic.

Another hypothesis attempts to explain the dementia by attributing it to a virus. According to this idea, some virus or virus-like agent may be responsible for initiating the disorder.

Evidence to support this notion has been presented. The type of neurofibrillary degeneration seen in AD has also been seen associated with a number of viral infections, including sub-acute sclerosing panencephalitis, multifocal leukonencephalitis, and postencephalitic Parkinson's disease. These researchers have not however, been able to produce in their experimental animals the type abnormalities so common in human AD, by means of infection.

One event that we know to be associated with infection is inflammation, which results in free-radical production, which in turn can lead to mitochondrial and cell damage. The fact that some AD-like neurodegeneration occurs with these infections may not so much be due to the infectious agent itself, but to the body's response to it, inflammation. If this is the so, then it may not so much be the disease that is the problem, but the treatment!

Another idea suggested is that neurons become damaged through neuroexcitation, a term used to describe a toxic reaction of the neuron to the natural chemical, glutamate, the primary excitatory neurotransmitter in the CNS. How can a neurotransmitter be toxic? The circumstance which turns glutamate from turning from friend to foe is a failure of cerebral respiration caused by atherosclerosis of the arteries supplying the brain, which in turn deprives the brain of oxygen, or from *respiratory collapse* of the mitochondria, or both. Glutamate activates a receptor on the surface of nerve cells known as the NMDA receptor. When this receptor is activated, Ca^{2+} rushes into the cell. Continual excitation of this receptor by glutamate would result in high levels of calcium inside the cell, and this, if not controlled, might lead to death of the neuron, because high levels of Ca^{2+} inside the cell is lethal.

Healthy individuals have a mechanism in their neurons and glial cells, which takes up the glutamate from the extracellular space, before it becomes poisonous. However, when you have low energy levels due to failure of respiration or ischemia, this important form of glutamate buffering cannot handle the load, because it depends on $Ca^{2+}/ATPase$ pumps, and these only work if you have sufficient ATP to drive them. Once NMDA-induced neuronal death begins to occur, microglia are attracted by the presence of stimuli provided by these lesioned neurons, and they in turn, contribute to the cell death, by attacking it as foreign, and through the release of ROS.

The circumstances, which raise our levels of oxidant stress, such as cerebral ischemia, inflammation and respiratory collapse, also cause an elevation of glutamate in the brain. The level of brain glutamate and ROS are intimately related. This is why the antioxidants vitamin E and GSH might protect cells from glutamate-induced cytotoxicity, because they interrupt the formation of the initiator, an abundance of ROS.

In many of these dementia-related conditions, you might have noticed two events seem to happen together. These are a build-up of glutamate, and a reduction in GSH. They occur together because they are related events. Glutamate normally is turned into GSH. This reaction also requires cysteine and ATP. If your levels of cysteine are low, because of some biochemical abnormality, or if insufficient ATP is present because of an uncoupling of oxidative phosphorylation, then you will not have the glutamate being used up by being incorporated into GSH, and you get an excess of this AA. An excess of glutamate, apart from being toxic, snowballs because it blocks cysteine uptake, which leads to even lower levels of GSH. It becomes a vicious cycle ending only in apoptotic death.

Treatment of cells in culture with stress (glucocorticoid) hormones stimulates cellular programmed death (apoptosis), and can bring about the type of apoptotic changes we been describing, involving the production of ROS and the depletion GSH. In this way, stress may be a contributor to these processes. This seems to be what happens to the cells of our thymus glands as we age. It appears that these cells undergo glucocorticoid-induced apoptotis, involving the particular pathways we have been discussing. This ultimately results in age-related atrophy of the thymus gland; or perhaps more honestly described as stress-related atrophy of the thymus gland, since these atrophic processes are more closely connected to stress, than to age.

Another thing that happens to us as we age is that a pigment called lipofuscin is deposited within cells. It is composed of peroxidized lipids and proteins. Although it has been observed in the olivery nucleus of infants, and in the spinal cord neurones of children, it accumulates progressively throughout our CNS as we age, especially in the cranial and spinal motor nuclei, the red nucleus, portions of the thalamus, and parts of the cerebellum. It is also found in the cerebral cortex, particularly in the large neurones of the precentral gyrus, and the cortical pyramidal cells.

Lipofuschin seems to accumulate in response to metabolic activity, rather than age. The type of metabolic activity with which it is most strongly related is oxidant enzyme activity. It is a side effect of metabolic stress, like the age spots that develop in the skin of some people with age. We do not know what consequences the accumulation of this pigment has for cellular function, but we do know that its accumulation can be reduced, at least in experimental animals by the dietary supplementation of antioxidants, such as vitamin E.

The brain is an organ that is working all the time. Like other organs it derives the energy for this work from respiration, but unlike other organs the brain is very susceptible to oxidant stress, not only because it is heavily respiring, but also because, it is largely made up of PUFAs, which are vulnerable to oxidation.

This situation is made worse by the fact that the defenses against oxidant damage are not very effective in the brain. A significant contributor to the symptoms of brain aging and dementia is this oxidant damage. Brain aging may be slowed to some extent by antioxidant-therapy, in particular those that are especially effective in this neural environment, reduced glutathione, vitamin E, melatonin and a Chinese herb called Gingko Biloba.

We must also remember to keep the brain active. Our brains are too smart to be idle. Having a brain as large as ours, and only using it for the basic functions of living, is like having a supercomputer in the basement, but only using it to generate the lotto numbers.

CHAPTER 8

FINDING THE NOBILITY WITHIN

Like the ocean is your godself, it remains undefiled,
and like the ether it lifts above the wind.
Even like the sun is your godself,
it knows not the ways of the mole,
nor seeks it the holes of the serpent

Kahlil Gibran, *The Prophet*

Can our emotions affect our physical health? It seems that almost everyone today has an opinion on this question. Many assertions are made on this without evidentiary support and presented as facts. The surfeit of pop psychology books published through the 1980s was, for the most part, merely expressing opinion. Let's now look at facts, and discover to what extent the mind can really influence physical health.

Firstly though, I need to tell you a story. David Spiegel was a psychiatrist associated with Stanford University working with women who had advanced breast cancer in the 1970s. If breast cancer is not treated early in its development, it can be very hard to treat. These women therefore had a poor prognosis. Spiegel was interested in the effect of *the healing web of mutual support.* He wanted to show that a support network could help people deal with emotional stress. His results were encouraging- he found such a support network could help the women cope with their situation.

About ten years later Spiegel reviewed his records to disprove a view fashionable in the 1980s, that one's emotions could alter the course of cancer. He could not. What he found was that those women who had been involved in the support groups survived twice as long as similarly placed, age-matched women, who had not had the advantages of emotional support. It only extended the lives of these women, not change the ultimate outcome, but it did suggest that the mind could have a bearing on physical disease.

The first inklings about the mind having a profound effect on the body occurred in 1974, and spawned a new science, psychoneuroimmunology (PNI). A psychologist, Robert Ader, was trying to run an experiment involving classical conditioning. Classical conditioning was the name of the practice used by Russian physiologist and Nobel laureate, Ivan Pavlov, who showed that dogs could be made to salivate upon hearing a bell, or seeing a flashing light, after they had associated that stimulus with the delivery of food. Ader was trying to teach rats to respond to saccharin-flavored water. He would give the rats the saccharin water and at the same time give them an injection of a drug, cyclophosphamide, to cause nausea. Normally, the rats would enjoy the saccharin water because it is sweet, but after associating it with the nausea caused by the cyclophosphamide it was hoped that they would learn, by classical conditioning, not to want it. They would have associated it with something unpleasant. This is called Aversion Conditioning.

The experiment did not go quite that way however. Ader found that many of his rats were dying, because the drug he was using to cause the nausea also suppressed the immune systems of the animals, causing them to get sick and die. Cyclophosphamide, he later discovered, apart from causing nausea, also lowers the number of T-lymphocytes, causing immunosuppression. What amazed Ader, and indeed the rest of the scientific world, was an accidental discovery he made. He found that when he gave animals that had been conditioned in this way the saccharin water alone, without the cyclophosphamide, their T-cell numbers still declined. This demonstrates in an elegant way the fact that it is not only animals that can learn, but that the immune system of these animals had apparently learned to associate the saccharin water with immunosuppression.

What was happening was that the brain of the animal was influencing its immune system. Up to this time that had never been thought possible. Clearly the rats did not know that cyclophosphamide would suppress their immune system, obviously there was some interaction, whereby the brain was associating the saccharin water with a suppressed immune system, and anticipating this effect. This experiment and others that followed it showed that there are connections between the immune system and the CNS, which hitherto had not been suspected.

Ader's discovery confirmed something physicians had known for a long time; the attitude of the patient can influence the outcome of their disease. This is the principle behind bedside manner. The idea dates back to that erudite Greek doctor, Hippocrates, who knew and taught that a physician's manner could be a medicine. But knowing and proving are two different things, and the 'proof' had to wait for Ader.

The stress response was designed by our evolution as a quick way for us to respond to infection, injury, or threat to our survival. However, today, for many of us, the stress response has become omnipresent. A little stress at the appropriate time is good for us. It helps us to focus and to survive. Chronic stress is not good for us. It suppresses the immune system, causes LDL to rise, causes our bones to lose calcium, can lead to high BP, headaches, diarrhea or other abdominal spasms, and increases the heart rate that can ultimately cause arrhythmias. What was intended by evolution to preserve us is now killing us.

Our minds can affect our immune system? Ader's first hard evidence of such a link in humans had focused the minds of the scientific community on the influence that mental events such as stress could have, on disease. PNI attracted many adherents.

These scientists started to look at other examples of where the immune system seemed to be modulated by mental events. Such examples started to tumble in. Astronauts had an altered immune function at the end of their missions; the immune system had been suppressed in people who had endured sleep deprivation, and also in others whose spouses had recently died. In all of these cases, suppression of the immune system was measured by recording the ways that the immune cells taken from these subjects would respond when stimulated. It was interesting and certainly suggestive of a relationship between stress and immunity, but it didn't measure whether or not these things would actually make people sick. The measuring was done in the test tube, in glass, or in vitro. What were needed were studies of the way things happen in nature, naturalistic studies. Later researchers conducted these, in 1991 for example, the New England Journal of Medicine published a seminal article that demonstrated a correlation between stress and susceptibility to the common cold.

Stress depresses the immune system. That is science! Often throughout history, there have been attempts to associate disease with personality characteristics, which we do not like. That is folklore! It is an attempt to blame the victim for the disease. Similar things were commonly said in relation to whatever was the world's most threatening disease from each epoch. Such comments were made about sufferers of TB during the 19th and early 20th centuries.

Today, you sometimes hear it said about cancer victims, and of course there was the AIDS epidemic of the 1980s, described by some as divine retribution. If you say that those with a disease have somehow brought it on themselves, by having qualities, which you denounce, then you reaffirm to yourself that this disease is not contracted by people like you.

Certain negative emotions however, can have a detrimental effect on our health. One is hostility. How does hostility do have this effect?

We know that the stress hormone adrenaline surges in hostile people. It is also thought that hostile people are more readily able to trigger the sympathetic nervous system, than are non-hostile individuals. The sympathetic nervous system and adrenaline both have the effect of speeding up one's heart rate. A continuously elevated heart rate, caused by being hostile, is like running your heart on benzene.

Under such conditions, there would be a higher level of oxidant stress, than would be found in the hearts of non-hostile people. Indeed studies have shown that animals which have high metabolic rates tend to have shorter life spans than those with low metabolic rates, unless they have the special protection of having low levels UFAs in their cell membranes. So it is very likely that oxidant stress is a factor in the pathology of hostility.

Whenever I hear about hostility and anger being a problem I think about the neurotransmitter serotonin. A high level of free-floating irrational anger suggests to me a deficiency of it. As well, a strong sympathetic response, a weak parasympathetic response, and increased eating, drinking and smoking characterize the so-called hostility syndrome. A recent study found that a high degree of repressed anger could be a risk factor for CHD, as it tends to lower HDL and raise LDL levels.

The more we examine the lipid connection with emotions the more intriguing it becomes. Our brains are largely composed of membranes, and membranes are largely composed of phospholipids.

A phospholipid consists of a long structure ending in a FA tail. In humans, the principal FA that comprises these FA tails is docosahexanoic acid (DHA). DHA is a FA common in fish oil. N-3 FAs such as DHA, are essential for the proper functioning of the brain. One recent finding showed that young men dosed with DHA, had a substantial reduction in the level of their aggression directed towards others at times of stress.

Can the emotions cause cancer? There are lots of books saying that positive thinking can cure cancers. What is usually common among these is the proposition that depression can lead to cancer. No such link has been established. There is a relationship between depression and a suppression of the immune response. People, who are taking selective serotonin reuptake inhibitor antidepressant drugs like Prozac™, get an augmentation of natural killer cell activity.

The natural killer cell is the Special Operations Commando of the immune system. People who are depressed, and those who are aging, often have relatively high levels of circulating cortisol (stress hormone) which we know, can suppress their immune system by reducing the numbers of circulating T-cells (lymphocytopenia), as well as the reactivity of those immune cells which are circulating.

One recent Italian study showed a higher volume of primary tumors among patients who had had stressful events in the six months before diagnosis, but the question of stress and cancer is far from clear. What is clear is the relationship investigated and proven by David Spiegel 20 years ago, that the best way for a cancer sufferer to extend his or her life is to have good social support. Love has healing qualities, which we do not fully understand.

Having successful relationships is important for good health. So is understanding the person closest in the world to you. The one who looks back at you from the mirror. Do you know that person? Do you understand that person? Because if you do not, you are living with a stranger, and that can be disastrous.

It is important to take some time out to find ourselves because it makes up for all the negative messages, which we receive about ourselves from others, and these messages are very destructive.

Guilt separates us from our own perfect spirituality, and as much as possible must be expunged from our consciousness.

A very large proportion of people today feel guilty about many things. We feel guilty, when we believe that we have not behaved in a way that is concordant with our inner codex of propriety. This codex, often called conscience, derives from many sources.

The nation state (and before that the tribe) hands down (sometimes inculcates) its mythology to us, included in which are a great number of stories designed to reinforce in us how someone of our tribe (or nation) should behave, what fundamental premises are important to our tribe, and therefore to us, the members. This forms the basis of the national/cultural mythology.

Although democracies such as the US, Australia, the UK and Western Europe are not overtly prescriptive in what its citizens should believe, under the surface at the level of a national mythology, the prescription is perceptible, and all the more powerful because it is covert, almost a national unconscious sea of shared-belief.

Another profound source of our personal mythology is the family. Children are not exactly born as a tabula rasa, a scraped tablet, upon which their parents and teachers merely write. Many future behavioral patterns are very much predetermined by the brain wiring, however, notwithstanding that, family does have a powerful impact. Most families have a myth teller. This could be a parent or someone more distantly related, who tells the child why it was that Uncle Frank died in the War. Most families have a Great Uncle who died in the War, and always have.

Certain organizations, which you might join have a mythology of their own, which gets superimposed on the existing mythologies that the individual has collected. One need only think of the US Marine Corps or the New York Police Department for examples of that sort of thing.

One of the most pervasive contributors to our personal mythology is religion. Perhaps one reason why it is such a powerful influence, is that this mythology is usually offered to us when we are very young. Often it is shared by our parents, who reinforce its validity. Sometimes it is inseparable from the national/cultural mythology, which also acts as a reinforcement, and often, deviation from the prescription contained within this transmitted wisdom is punished by group ostracism, disgrace and/or eternal torture.

Priests, pastors, rabbis, and imams work on us from an early age, propounding what we must do, but more especially, what we must not do. To deviate from the mythological prescription is described as sin, and sin we are told, or at least I was by Irish Catholic priests, is a terrible thing. Something likely to bring disgrace to our parents, and an eternity in hellfire to us.

So where does the word sin come from? This wretched word, which has caused so many of us, a lifetime shackled to unpleasant feelings of guilt and unworthiness. It may not surprise you to hear that it comes from the Bible, but what might surprise you is that it is actually a mistranslation. The word sin is derived from the Greek word sunde and the Latin word sons, which means guilty.

The Bible, of course, was translated into Greek and Latin from Hebrew. The word for which sin is supposed to be a translation, was in the original Hebrew word hamartia. However this does not mean guilt at all. It actually means to fall short of perfection, or to miss the mark. In short, it means to make a mistake. Now we've all made mistakes haven't we? Nothing to get your knickers in a knot about!

This mistranslation of a fairly mild Hebrew word into one with all sorts of dire connotations has served one group well. That group is the professional religious celebrant, or office holder. We call them priests, pastors, rabbis and imams, and the thing, which has engaged the energy of these people the most, is sexuality.

One of the most common things that people feel guilty about is their sexuality. Sexuality is our second most powerful drive after self-preservation, and it is really something! Almost irresistible! It has to be, the continuation of the species depends upon it. For most of us, it is there noticeably lurking in the background most of the time, while we go about our business, trying to do other things. We have learned as part of our national/cultural mythology, that there are only certain acceptable situations where it can be brought to the foreground, and most of us observe these strictures. During our 20s, when we are at the height of our powers, we think of little else. Later, it is still there, with us all, the time, like a personal dragon, which we have learned to tame, but only to a point.

The priests, pastors, rabbis and imams seem to be obsessed with sexuality and many of their harshest prescriptions are reserved for it. Why is that! It always seemed more than passing strange to me that a Creator God would go to all the trouble of creating sexuality, as a very powerful drive, and then tell everyone that it was forbidden. Who said that God doesn't have a sense of humor?

Well, of course that is not what happened. The priests, pastors, rabbis and imams tell us the sex is prohibited, except under certain rigidly prescribed circumstances, such as a church-sanctioned marriage. Why do they say this? Because it gives them control over our lives.

A person's sexuality is at his or her core. You can think of a person as being like an onion-you peel away the outer layers and there is another layer inside, and as soon as you peel away that one, you reveal another. Eventually, you will get to the point where you can not peel any more layers away; you reach the kernel; the solid nub at the center of the human onion. This is human sexuality. The very core of a person. Control that, and you control the individual. This is why priests, pastors, rabbis, and imams (or to be more correct the organizations which they represent) are so interested in it. It all boils down to a matter of control.

What should religion really be about? The word religion is derived from re-ligare, the Latin word meaning re-tie or reconnect. What religion is really about is the reconnection of us with our own spirituality, It is not really about control. It is about finding your own Spirit, not finding someone to tell you what you can or cannot do.

As we enter the third millennium, it's time to put away childish things. Although religion is not without its negative consequences, some of them grave ones, I think on the whole its effect on human society has been positive. But hey! Now we've grown up. Now the time has arrived where we can begin to think for ourselves, to put away the mythology, and to experience the reality of spirituality, which powers this grand and beautiful Universe for ourselves. To find God not without but within, and in everything around us.

In order to do this, we need to spend some time with ourselves. We need to be quiet enough, long enough, to hear the Universe talking to us. You do not necessarily have to be alone. You can be with other people as long as you are quiet and vigilant, not tense, aware, creatively aware; listening to what the Universe has to say to you. It often helps to be in a natural setting for this sort of dialogue, in the forest, by the sea or in the mountains, somewhere where the full majesty of the Universe can easily impinge on your consciousness.

In these quiet times, when it is just you and the Universe, you should reflect on what type of person is the one who bears your name? What is he or she looking for out of life, and why? What does he or she like doing, and why? If all the answers do not come at once, don't let that discourage you. Sometimes the Universe is mute while she determines if this is a serious enquiry or not. Eventually though, the answers will come. Just keep asking those questions. Reflect on the things you feel guilty about in particular and try to understand them and their impact on you. You are aiming to discover yourself. You need to understand your role in life, no matter how modest it might at first seem.

In order to explain why you should do this, I refer to one of the greatest books in the world's literature, The Bagavadgita. This work is a part of a larger work called the Mahabharata, a great epic, which forms part of the astonishingly rich Indian Vedic literature, and which contains all that one needs to know about life, death and resurrection, in all of its manifestations.

The Bagavadgita is essentially a dialogue between Arjuna a warrior, and his charioteer Krishna. Arjuna finds himself reluctantly involved in a civil war, and on the eve of the battle, he expresses to Krishna his feelings of guilt (sin) and remorse about his having to kill people that he knows. Krishna's response is that Arjuna is a warrior, and such he has the role of a warrior.

We all have roles in life. We just have to find them, and when people do find their roles, they at last feel complete. That is the message in the 3500 year old Vedic bottle. Think about it!

The attitude that you take to sin is your own business, but sin is not a religious idea. Sin is an ethical concept that has nothing to do with religion-real religion, that is. Real religion has no place for a list of pre-scribed and proscribed behavior. The correct place for such concerns is in philosophy, or even the law, but not religion.

Understand that you do not have to beat yourself up anymore. Indeed you must not do that! We are not fallen angels, as first Judaic then its offspring, Christian and Islamic tradition, maintained. That was a story for human society during its infancy. The overall effect of it has been to keep us like little children. In the Third Millennium, we can be grown-up about our spirituality, and an important part of being grown up is taking responsibility for yourself. This means forgiving yourself, and accepting, nay encouraging, your part in this Universe, the vast perpetually unfolding cloth of many colors.

Aging does not have to arouse fear. It can be an exciting time. A time when one is at one's peak. After a lifetime of experience, a character is now in full bloom. The Greek philosopher Heraclitus said: "*Character is fate.*" These are wise words, because our character is the currency by which we negotiate our lives, and form and maintain relationships. Nothing can be more pertinent to the safe conduct of one's life than character, and as we get old we are given the time we are given to distill and purify our characters. If we employ the character-refining role of aging appropriately, we can find it very satisfying, leading to a more ful-filled life. We can find that being free, to some degree at least, of the constant nagging to reproduce, or at least to have sex, a situation that Sophocles the ancient Greek

dramatist described as: *a great relief,* we have the time to work on ourselves in a way we never could when we were younger. With aging, it is possible to get wisdom.

The End

INDEX

A

Acetyl Coenzyme A, 33
Actin, 37, 66
Active transport, 31
Advanced gkycation end products
    (AGEs), 65
Aging
    and metabolic rate, 81
    and brain shrinkage, 182
Alcohol
    and brain damage, 204
Aluminum
    and dementia, 204
Alzheimer, 187
Alzheimer's disease
    and homocysteine, 205
Anaerobic glycolysis, 28
Andropause (male 'menopause'),
55
Anger
    and heart disease, 112
Antioxidant defenses, 68-69
Antioxidant vitamins, 69
Antioxidants and cancer, 145
Archeon Epoch, The, 15
Aspirin
    and cancer, 147
Atherosclerosis, 88-90
ATP, 32

B

Back pain, 177-78
Benign tumors, 116

Benzene, 65
Beta amyloid, 185, 195-7
Beta-carotene, 69
Bioflavonoid, 95
Blood pressure and heart disease,
108
Body Mass Index (BMI), 105
Bone
    types of, 150-51
    cells of, 152
Brain aging
    and glutathion, 192
Brain damage
    and alcohol, 204
    and respiratory collapse, 197-
201
Brain shrinkage, 182
Breast cancer, 132-36
    and estrogen, 124
    and fish consumption, 135
    and nuns, 124

C

Calcitonin, 156
Cancer
    and aspirin, 147
    and inflammation, 146
    and viruses, 127
    a multistep process, 123
    cockroaches and the Nobel
Prize, 149
    communities with low levels
        of, 124

definition of, 116
of the breast, 132-36
of the colon, 128-131
of the cervix (of the uterus), 138
primary protection strategy, 148-149
Carbon Cycle, The, 17
Cataracts, 52
Cell divisions
number of, 120
Cell membrane failure, 64
Cellulose, 35
Cerebral ischemia, 188
Cholesterol
and the cell membrane, 74
and the heart, 91
CML, 76
Coenzyme Q$_{10}$, 47-49
Colon cancer, 128-31
Coronary Heart Disease
incidence of, 83
risk factors, 85
Cruciferous vegetables, 132
Cytomegalovirus and heart disease, 90
Cytoskeleton
damage to, 66-68, 77

D

Darwin and Wallace, 25
Dementia, 185
Dementia
and aluminium, 204
and viruses, 205
decrease in glycolysis, 195
Digital divide, 50
Diseases of aging
throughout history, 55-56

Diverticulosis, 52
DNA
Origins, 20
oxidant damage of, 78-80

E

Endothelium, 85
Essential fatty acids, 131, 135
and breast cancer, 135, 136
and cancer metasasies, 138
and curtailment of aggression, 213
and heart disease, 59, 98
and osteoarthritis, 173, 177, 179
in the prevention of cancer, 135, 137
Evolution by Natural Selection, 25
Exercise
and breast cancer, 134
and heart disease, 109
and oxidant stress, 71-72

F

Fats
and cancer, 135
and chronic degenerative diseases, 136
and disease, 59
Fatty acids, 41-45
Fatty streak, 94
Fermentation, 36
Fish consumption
and curtailment of aggresion, 213
and breast cancer, 135, 136
and heart disease, 59, 98
and osteoarthritis, 173, 177, 179

Foam cell, 94
Folate and heart disease, 104-105
Free radicals
    a cause of disease, 45, 60, 64
    and cellular energy failure, 65
    and membrane receptor
        proteins, 65
    and mitochondrial damage ,
        68
    causing brain damage, 191-
        94, 200
    causing cell nucleus damage,
        78, 80
    damage done by, 62
    failure of membrane ion
        pumps, 65
    generated by peroxidized
        lipids, 75
    in osteoarthritis, 174
    in physical exercise , 71
    in prostaglandin synthesis, 62
    in the respiratory burst, 93
    numbers of in cigarette
        smoke, 66
    produced by cytochromes, 62
    produced by the immune
        system, 62, 93, 138, 146
    produced by liver detoxification,
        62
    what are they? 61
French Paradox, 72, 96
Functional reserve capacity
    of the brain, 195

G

George Washington, 96
Globalization, 50-51
Glutathione, 69
    and cervical cancer , 139

and brain aging, 192
Glycocalyx, 40
Glycoproteins, 34, 40
Greenhouse Effect, The
    on the early Earth, 15, 17

H

HDL, 90, 99-101
Heart disease
    incidence of, 83
    risk factors, 85
    and anger, 112
    and bacteria, 90
    and blood pressure, 108
    and exercise, 109
    and the oral contraceptive
pill, 101
    and stress, 111
    and your job, 114
    primary prevention, 110-11
Helicobacter pylori, 52
Hiatus hernia, 52
Hip fractures, 162
Homoccysteine
    and atherosclerois, 103
    and heart disease, 86, 88, 98
    causes damage to the
endothelium, 104
    counteracted by folate, 104
    in Alzheimer's disease, 205
    interferes wit blood clotting,
        103-04
    safe in the liver, 102
Hormone Replacement Therapy
(HRT), 164-66
Hostility, 113
Hydroxyl radical, 62, 65, 67, 68,
    70

I

Inflammation
and the brain,193, 202, 205
and cancer, 146
and heart disease, 87-90
Insulin, 36, 37

K

Ketosis, 39
Kidney stones
and calcium supplementa-
tion, 164

L

Laws of Thermodynamics, 22
Life-span energy potential, 81
Lipid peroxidation and aging, 74
Lipofuschin, 81
in the brain, 207
Low density lipoprotein (LDL),
91-94
Lung cancer, 141

M

Male 'menopause,' 55
Malignant tumors, 117
Meat-eating
in the pre-history of humans,
58
Melatonin, 81
Membrane fluidity, 73-74
Membrane ion pumps
and oxidant stress, 65
Menopause, 52-54
The 'Granny' theory of, 54
Miller and Urey, experimenters,
16-18

Mind and the immune system,
211
Mitochondria
abnormalities of cause
ischemia, 48
acquistion of, 29
and cerebral ischemia, 188
coenzyme Q_{10} in, 47
cytochromes in, 63
death throws of, 199-200
efficiency of oxidation in, 44
damage to their DNA, 78
190-91
electron leakage in, 63
fatty acids oxidized in, 44
highly susceptible to
oxidative damage, 67
number of , 78
oxidative phosphorylation in,
45
proton pump of, 47
respiration in, 36
Respiratory Collapse in, 189,
199
source of free radicals, 62
structure of, 40
Mitochondrial Medicine, 29
Monosaccharides, 34-35
Motor-vehicle emissions
and childhood asthma, 66
Mutagenic Potential, 146

N

Neuronal plasticity, 183
N-nitrosamine, 139

O

Oil of gladness, 41
Olive oil
    and cancer protection, 137
Oncogene, 125-127
Oparin, Alexksandr, 16

Oral contraceptive pill
    and breast cancer, 133
    and heart disease, 101
Osteoarthritis, 169
    and heredity, 172
    and inflammation, 173
oxidant deterioration of collagen,
174, 176-7
Osteoporosis
    and calcium supplementation,
    159
    and cigarette smoking, 155,
    160
    and genetics, 160
    and insulin-like growth factors,
    157
    and magnesium, 157-58
    and physical inactivity, 168
    causes of, 157
    in males and females, 155
    throughout history, 162-63
Osteoporotic fractures, 161-62
Oxidant stress, 61
    and brain damage, 189-192
    and lifespan, 61
    and Parkinson's disease, 202
Oxidative phosphorylation, 45-47

P

P_{450} detoxification pathway, 132

p53
    gene, 120, 128
    protein, 119
Pap smear, 138
Papillomas, 122
Periodontal disease, 52
Pernicious anemia, 52
Peroxidized lipids
    the oxidative effect of, 75
Phenolics, 95- 97
Photosynthesis
    origins of, 27
Phytoestrogems , 134
Polyphenols, 72, 95
Positron Emission Tomography,
    194
Presbyacusis, 52
Prostacyclin I_2, 86
Prostaglandins, 44, 86
Proteins, 19, 37
Psychoneuroimmunology, 210

R

Radical oxygen species (ROS), 61
Respiratory burst, 93
Respiratory collapse, 189
Rickets, 155

S

Salt and high blood pressure, 60
Saltatory conduction, 41
Schwann cell, 40-41
Selenium
    and heart disease, 98
    overdose of, 99
Smoking
    and heart disease, 106-107
    and oxidant stress, 66
Stomach cancer, 139

Stress
    and heart disease, 111
 · and the immune system, 212
Sudden death, 114
Superoxide, 63
Superoxide dismutase, 69

T

Tea, 72
Tumor
    Promotors, 122
    suppressor gene, 128, 144
Tungusta Event, The, 18

V

Vasoactive amines, 86
Viruses and cancer, 127
Vitamin A, 71
Vitamin C, 71
Vitamin D, 155
Vitamin E, 70

X

Xenobiotics, 65